Alkaline

2 Books in 1

Alkaline Fasting to Lose Fat, Increase Your Spirituality and Heal Your Body from Within

Table of Contents

Alkaline Diet

One Meal a Day Intermittent Fasting

Alkaline Diet

Ultimate Guide for Beginners - Naturally Lose Weight, Reverse Disease and Gain Unlimited Energy

J.P. Edwin

professional before attempting any techniques outlined in this book.

By reading this document, the reader agrees that under no circumstances is the author responsible for any losses, direct or indirect, which are incurred as a result of the use of information contained within this document, including, but not limited to, — errors, omissions, or inaccuracies.

Introduction

Over the past years, there have been a number of different diet plans introduced into the market. Some of these diet plans have managed to make a big impact while others faded within a few months of gaining popularity.

When it comes to weight loss, people often look for the more convenient methods to get fit rather than something that can benefit the body. If you want to lose weight, then your main motto shouldn't just be to burn fat but also to get healthy and prevent the risk of a number of diseases from occurring. You have to follow a healthy diet plan that works well on your body and mind, and also helps you stay healthy by lowering the risk of some of the most chronic illnesses which people suffer from when they do not pay attention to their health.

The reason an alkaline diet has gained so much popularity is because it focuses not only on weight loss but on decreasing the risk of diseases that are caused due to lack of nutrients and antioxidants in the body. The diet plan that Dr. Sebi introduced not only managed to prove effective when applied to your daily lifestyle, but it also turned out to be an easy diet plan to follow as soon as your body got used to it.

This detailed guide gives you hands-on information about an alkaline diet, what you need in order to follow the diet, and how it can benefit you with a few changes in your lifestyle. You will also understand why Dr. Sebi encourages people to adapt to veganism. This guide will help you transform your mind body and soul!

Chapter 1 - What Is Alkalinity? Why Should I Care?

It's no hidden secret that certain foods work well on your body while others have bad side effects. But the key to understanding which food is healthy for you and what kind of food you need to avoid is important because in between a burger and a salad, there is a lot of room for you to introduce healthier options that can help your body heal from within and make you look great at the same time.

The one factor that helps you to understand how healthy you are is figuring out whether you have an alkaline body or an acidic body. If you have a high acidic level, then you need to understand how you can alkalize your body to lead a healthy lifestyle.

When you suffer from high acidic levels in your body, you are more prone to problems such as fatigue or low energy levels. Other signs of high acid levels in your body also include brittle nails and hair. It is also known to cause low bone density and osteoporosis in women which can cause multiple fractures with a simple fall. Although people do not take acidic levels in their body that seriously - and they should, it also results in heavy breathing and weight gain, which is often followed by obesity. An acidic diet can also introduce digestive issues along with diabetes. People with high acidic levels are also known to suffer from skin related problems and acne, and have a low immune system which means they are more susceptible to infections and allergies. These people are also at a higher risk of heart problems and cancer. If you want to stay away from these problems, it's important for you to transform your body into an alkaline body by following a healthy diet.

What Is Alkalinity?

An alkaline diet is based on the content of alkalinity in your body. Your alkalinity levels are measured by figuring out whether you have higher alkaline content or higher acidic content in your body. While the total alkalinity in your body means having a high pH level, the truth is while pH levels are a part of an alkaline diet, it does not make up the diet completely. For instance, alkalinity in a body is measured by the amount of Alkaline substances present in the water content in your body. The normal pH level for alkalinity is anything between 0 to 14. If you have a pH level that is higher than 7, your body is neutral and if it's lower than 7, this means you have more acidic content in your system.

Anything above 7 indicates higher alkalinity levels while below 7 indicates acidic levels in the body. It is important for every person to understand the level of alkalinity in the body because a diet plan is to be based on the pH level of the individual. If your pH levels are very low, you need to make sure you stay away from acidic food and also make sure that you consume nutritious foods. Most people today have high acidic content in the system which is why focusing on an alkaline diet is something you need to consider doing. Foods such as meat and fresh dairy, eggs, grain, and alcohol all contain high acidic levels that aren't great for the body. Neutral foods are usually natural fats, sugar and starches which also need to be avoided. An alkaline diet is basically a diet that is filled with fruits, legumes, and vegetables. These are the kind of foods you need to focus on eating to get healthy.

What Exactly Does "pH Level" Mean?

The term pH is not new and you have probably heard it numerous times in your classroom during a science class. The pH scale is basically used to measure the alkalinity or acidity in any substance where 7 is considered to be the neutral number and anything above it is alkaline where is anything below it is acidic. To measure the alkalinity or acidity in a substance, you need an aqueous solution. Human blood is aqueous because it contains high water content and this means that there is a pH level in your blood as well. This doesn't mean you can test the pH level in your blood because the pH level in your blood will not change except for when you are in a critical situation and have a life-threatening disease.

The alkaline levels in your saliva and urine however keep changing depending on the kind of food that you eat, and this enables you to understand your cellular health. The reason this is important is because without monitoring the cellular level, you will not manage to figure out whether you are healthy or not.

While the pH levels in your blood usually clock under 7, the levels in urine could go as low as 3. To begin following a healthy alkaline diet, you need to understand how long your levels of alkalinity are. This will help you figure out what needs to be changed and how you have to make the changes.

The reason monitoring your pH levels is important is because when it goes considerably low, your body turns acidic and you could even suffer from something known as chronic low-grade acidosis. This is normally caused when there is a high consumption of acidic foods that impact your body and results in low calcium, potassium, magnesium, and mineral levels in your body.

Research has proven that following an alkaline diet can help reduce multiple health-related problems and aid in effective weight loss. This is why it's important for you to understand how the pH levels in your body impact your overall health.

What Is The Alkaline Diet?

An alkaline diet is a diet that helps lower the acidic levels in your body by maintaining the pH balance. Therefore you lose weight and get healthier, lowering the risk of multiple diseases. This diet had gained a lot of popularity when Dr. Sebi openly spoke about how effective it is and how incorporating the diet plan into your daily routine can help you lead a longer and more fruitful life.

Figuring out an alkaline diet could cause a lot of confusion because this diet may seem very complicated when you take a glance. In theory, an alkaline diet is a diet that helps lower your body"s acidic levels. This may seem like a bit tough to understand but when you start consuming fruits that have higher alkaline content and lower acidic content, it is obvious that your body starts healing. This will make it come closer to a healthy alkaline level rather than an acidic one. There are tons of food that reduce a lot of acid in your body and people are so used to consuming these foods on a regular basis, they don't realize what's affecting their body. Following a regular diet plan may seem like the perfect solution because it reflects on your weighing scale and you even notice that you have lost a few pounds. However, that doesn't necessarily mean you are getting any healthier. If you want to stay healthy, you have to lower the risk of diseases in your system and keep your vital organs functioning effectively. That's what an alkaline diet does to you which is why once people understand how effective the diet plan is, they start adapting towards leading an alkaline lifestyle and avoiding foods that have high acidic content.

Testing Yourself For Acidity

Once you have decided you want to follow the alkaline diet, you need to start planning the small changes in your lifestyle one step at a time. Taking a plunge into the first diet plan you see is not the ideal solution because everybody is different and for you to make the most out of this diet plan, you need to understand your pH level before you move forward. To do this, you need to test your acid levels and see just how high the acidic level is.

Testing for acidic levels in your body is very simple. You need to get a pH test paper. This paper tests the acid and alkaline levels of any liquid and you can either use urine or saliva to test your acidic levels. However, it is highly recommended that you test it with the first urine you collect in the morning after at least 6 hours of uninterrupted sleep. To do the test, all you need to do is take a strip of the paper and dip it into a cup of urine you have accumulated or urinate directly on the paper. If you are not comfortable urinating, you can then spit on the paper as soon as you get up in the morning.

When you purchase the pH paper, it comes with a color chart to help you figure out just how acidic or basic your body is. The colors usually range from yellow to blue and they have numbers written by their side. As mentioned earlier, if you are below seven, it means you are on the acidic side but if you are above 7, you are healthy.

There is more sense to purchase the pH test paper and use it every now and then. The reason being once you incorporate the diet plan you will manage to measure results on a regular basis and this helps keep your motivation levels high.

Signs Your Body Is Too Acidic

While it may be easy to get pH testing paper from various shopping websites all over the internet, in case you haven't managed to find this test strip yet, you can always look out for the early warning signs. These signs will tell if your body is too acidic and you need to take charge for you to live a healthy life.

1. One of the major signs that your body is too acidic is when you start feeling too tired even if you've rested for over 8 hours every night. People who have a high acid content in their system tend to feel tired and low on energy even with enough rest.

2. High acidic levels in your body also make you feel sad and depressed most of the time. Even it is a reason to celebrate and you still can't feel genuinely happy, this could be a sign that you have high acidic levels in your body.

3. People who suffer from high acidic levels also tend to get irritable for no apparent reason and they snap very easily. If you are told that you are snappy or irritable, this

could be because you have high acidic levels.

4. Another common sign that you have high acidic levels is the inability to focus effectively on your task. If you find it difficult to get your mind in one place and get a job done effectively, this is another sign that your acidic levels are high and it needs to be brought down under control.

5. Low immunity levels and the susceptibility to infections such as cold and flu is another common sign of a high acidic level.

6. People who also suffer from skin problems and dry skin, even during warmer months of the year, could have a high acidic level.

7. Hormonal imbalance is another sign that you need to be on the lookout for.

8. Another common problem involves digestive issues which could be a combination of constipation along with diarrhea.

9. Shortness of breath, chronic pain, sensitivity in teeth and gums and a stiff neck are also common signs that your body is too acidic and you need to do something to change it.

These are some of the early signs and the sooner you identify them, the better it is because you will manage to shift towards a healthy diet plan.

Chapter 2 - Who Was Dr. Sebi?

Dr. Sebi happens to be the inspiration behind the alkaline diet. He was known to be a herbalist and intracellular therapist and a natural healer who was native to Honduras. His diet is inspired by his native land and includes a ton of alkaline foods which are natural and help curb the side effects of high acidic levels in the body.

He designed the diet plan after extensive research and understanding how much trouble acidic levels caused to the body, and why it's necessary to protect the body against acid levels and mucus, that later develop into various diseases. His teachings have managed to enrich the lives of many and helped them to promote healthy living. The alkaline diet plan he came up with not only paved the path toward healing the most life-threatening diseases, but also helped to control the risk related to those diseases. It also helped people to cope with the disease more effectively. The alkaline diet not only works well for weight loss but it has also proven to be beneficial in curing diseases such as diabetes, epilepsy, lupus, cancer, and even HIV.

The main focus of Dr. Sebi"s diet was to reduce the amount of acidic foods you consume because this helps to make it difficult for diseases to thrive in your body. Dr. Sebi invested over 40 years researching how alkaline foods can promote healthy living and he finally came up with a diet plan that works well not only to lose weight but to heal your system from within.

History

Dr. Sebi led a controversial life, and a number of people believed his teachings were not beneficial in any way. He was bold enough to come out in the open and say that he can find the cure to deadly diseases like cancer, AIDS, and diabetes that hadn"t been found after all the years of medical research. His main motto was to convince people to lead a healthy life and understand the importance of alkaline foods in the regular diet.

Dr. Sebi received a lot of backlash and people believed he was trying to dupe them and force them to lead a vegan life. But once he made people understand just how effective his methods were, not only did he gain celebrity following but he also became one of the most popular herbalists you could find.

Amongst the various accusations Dr. Sebi had against him, there was one that went up to the Supreme Court. This accusation was against an advertisement he released in 1988 for claiming to cure people of deadly diseases. The court believed they had a strong case and they wanted to put him away. However, a staggering 77 people came into the court saying that they were cured after following Dr. Sebi"s advice and incorporating his food into their lifestyle. As per the witnesses, 77 people declared he was not guilty and they also proved that his diet plan turned out to be a medical miracle and he was underrated.

Life moved on and people never forgot about Dr. Sebi and what an amazing healer he was. All his life he tried to make as many people understand the importance of an alkaline diet so that they could keep their diseases away.

Philosophy On Eating Natural Foods

According to Dr. Sebi, there is a wide variety of plant-based food that you should focus on eating. Although he believes veganism is a smart way to get rid of all your health problems, he does not force you to follow such a diet. The core focus of this alkaline diet is that you eat natural and healthy foods, which enables your body to lower the acidic level and helps you heal from within.

The main philosophy of adopting an alkaline diet is so that your metabolic system starts functioning effectively once again. When your body has high contents of acid inside of it, it affects the metabolic system and this means that your body uses most of the food that you eat to be stored as fat rather than convert it into energy. When your acid levels are right at the top, it is difficult for your metabolism to work effectively and this causes a problem with the overall digestive system. If you want to start living a healthy life, you have to begin eating food that works to enhance digestion for your bodily functions to work systematically. The first stage is for your metabolism to start increasing and to convert the food you eat into energy rather than storing it in your body as fat.

When you start eating healthy foods, your pH level starts balancing out. This process takes time but it slowly and surely gets you leaning towards an alkaline way of life which benefits you in the long run. The philosophy of natural food is to ensure that you do not skip meals to lose weight but rather to include foods that are high in calcium and magnesium as well as natural fat in order to alkalize your body. There are a number of benefits you get when you follow a healthy natural diet and this not only reflects in your appearance but you also start feeling a lot better.

Veganism

It's no secret that alkaline diet promotes veganism and encourages people to go vegan so that they can stay healthy. Although it is recommended to become a vegan while you follow the alkaline diet, it's not compulsory and if your body can handle a little meat and milk, there is no reason for you to stop consuming it completely. However, controlling the amount of non-vegetarian food items you include can help you to keep a healthy heart and have a ton of other benefits, which is why it is recommended in the alkaline diet.

Apart from the obvious reasons in helping alkalize your body, veganism is also beneficial in various other ways.

Here are a few reasons why doctors believe veganism is a healthy lifestyle.

Rich In Nutrients

Although a lot of people believe that non-vegetarian food items are high in protein and can manage to provide your body with all the necessary nutrients required to keep the body healthy, veganism is actually healthy and is based on the nutrient levels of food.

When you consume a high non-vegetarian diet, the only thing you are providing your body with is protein. A vegan diet, on the other hand, comprises of whole foods that not only include high levels of fiber and antioxidants but also contain Vitamin A, C, E, B and Folic acids as well as potassium and magnesium.

If you want your vegan diet to work in your favor, you need to check the nutrient content of every meal you consume to make sure you give your body everything that it needs. While vegan diets are high in antioxidants and Vitamin E and C, you also need to have enough iron and calcium intake so that you get stronger bones. There are tons of vegan food that are high in iron and banana is a classic example.

It Helps In Weight Loss

A number of people who suffer from obesity and weight issues are usually non-vegetarian. They have a higher content of fat in comparison to a vegan diet. If you follow a controlled diet and ensure you eat right, you will manage to lose weight faster compared to any other diet plan you choose to follow. When you combine veganism with an alkaline diet, not only does it boost your weight loss process, it also helps you to feel better and regularizes your blood sugar level thereby lowering the risk of diabetes.

Low Risk Of Cancer

According to the World Health Organisation, controlling what you eat plays a huge role in lowering the risk of cancer. Acidic foods and non-vegetarian foods are right at the top of high-risk foods. They are more prone to causing cancer in comparison to fresh fruits and vegetables which are consumed by vegans on a regular basis.

Lowers The Risk Of Heart Disease

Vegan are less prone to heart conditions and heart diseases in comparison to those who do not follow a vegan diet. The cholesterol level in a vegan is always lower than one who eats meat, and cholesterol is one of the leading reasons for heart-related problems. This is why a vegan diet is highly recommended if you have high cholesterol levels. Vegans also consume a lot of whole grains which work extremely well in promoting good heart health.

Reduces Arthritis Pain

If you suffer from arthritis, then probiotic rich and raw vegan food can work wonders to lower the painful effect that it causes. Based on recent research, people who switched from a non-vegetarian diet to a natural whole food vegan diet for a span of 6 weeks managed to note a higher energy level and better functionality in comparison to other arthritis patients. The diet helps in greatly reducing joint swelling and stiffness, including pain that is common with rheumatoid arthritis and joint pain.

Before you plan a vegan diet, you need to understand that there are various kinds of foods in the diet plan which you should and shouldn't include. To figure out which food is healthy for you and which is not, you have to learn the alkaline content in the food. Vegan foods that have high acidic content should always be avoided because this is not going to benefit your body in any way. While vegan food is good, combining it with an alkaline diet is what plays a key role in helping you lose weight and fighting off diseases effectively.

Chapter 3 - Benefits Of Alkalinity

An alkaline diet is all about increasing the alkalinity in your body to help you lead a healthy and long life that's disease free. This diet plan has been making waves in the market because of the effectiveness that it has to offer and more and more people are now planning to get used to the diet plan.

One of the major reasons why the alkaline diet has gained so much popularity is because it helps people get slim; however, that's not the only thing that alkalinity can help you with. Once you understand how alkalinity works and what it does to your body, you will never want to switch back to a diet plan that contains a high acid content.

Protects Bone Density and Muscle Mass

Research has proven that high acid content in your body can affect your bones as well as your muscles. The reason it is important for you to focus on alkaline meals is because it increases the mineral intake in your body and focuses on better bone structure, resulting in lesser brittle bones. The acid content in your body is responsible for bone problems including joint pain and arthritis. When you lower the acid contents in your body, it gets easier for your bones to become stronger and absorb the healthy minerals that contribute towards better bone health. An alkaline diet focuses on increasing the production of vitamin D absorption in the bone and this is responsible for keeping your bones healthy. It also helps in the production of growth hormone and in ensuring that your body gets more strength from the minerals consumed. This helps effectively increase muscle mass and strength.

By increasing the alkalinity in your body, not only do you get better bones and better muscle strength but your endurance increases and you manage to exercise more effectively. This is vital for your overall health and it helps to keep away a number of bone-related diseases. When you have strong muscles, your body stays firmer and you age more gracefully.

Lowers Risk for Hypertension and Stroke

Following an alkaline diet has a lot of anti-aging effects on the body. Apart from helping to protect muscle mass, it also decreases inflammation in the body and this works well to relieve a lot of stress and enhances cardiovascular health. People who follow an alkaline diet are less prone to hypertension and cholesterol. One of the leading causes of stroke is high cholesterol levels and blood clots caused by this cholesterol content. When you start an alkaline diet, your cholesterol level falls into place and it also helps to regulate blood pressure which is responsible for hypertension.

When you relieve stress, you start leading a healthy life not only physically but mentally as well. Stress is directly related to memory loss and a number of brain-related illnesses including Alzheimer's disease and Dementia. When you consume an alkaline based diet, you lower the risk of these diseases, and also prevent the risk of a heart attack and high blood pressure.

Alkaline-based diets also work really well on your vital organs including your kidneys. Kidney stones can be excruciatingly painful. One of the major causes of kidney stone is the acid content in your body and when this content is reduced, you lower the risk.

Lowers Chronic Pain and Inflammation

It's no secret that some women suffer from severe menstrual cramps during their menstruation while others manage to handle it more effectively. The leading cause of cramps during menstruation is high acid levels in the body. When you begin following an alkaline based diet, you reduce the risk of suffering from painful cramps because it helps soothe the muscles and relax them.

Alkalinity also helps prevent chronic back pain, muscle spasms, headache, inflammation, and joint pains. By simply reducing the acid levels in your body, you can keep a number of these problems at bay. When your body is healthier, you have more energy and you are able to get a lot more done during the day. It is important for you to have relaxed muscles and keep away inflammation and chronic pain to start leading a healthy lifestyle. This is where alkalinity comes into the picture and this is why it's so important.

Boosts Vitamin Absorption and Prevents Magnesium Deficiency

Magnesium deficiency is highly underrated and people don't understand the importance of getting adequate magnesium in your body. When you fail to provide your body with the right amount, a lot of enzymes in your system begin dysfunctioning and it's not possible for your body to carry out its regular processes effectively. Lack of magnesium is one of the main causes of heart diseases and muscle spasms. It is also responsible for headache, sleep anxiety, and insomnia. When your magnesium levels are optimum, it also helps in activating Vitamin D and boosts the absorption of this vitamin into your bones for healthier and stronger bones. Magnesium also works well with other vitamins and helps the body get the benefits of those vitamins by absorbing it more effectively.

Helps Improve Immune Functionality and Cancer Protection

One of the major benefits of alkalinity is that it helps oxidize your body more effectively and dispose of waste material faster. Apart from helping boost your metabolism level, it also strengthens the immune system to get rid of the dirty toxins on a regular basis. When you have a stronger immune system, your body manages to fight off bacteria and infections better. An alkaline diet contains high antioxidant properties responsible for fighting off the free radical cells mainly responsible for cancer cells growing in the system. An alkaline diet can help reduce the risk of cancer by killing these cells.

People who have multiple health problems should move to an alkaline based diet because not only does this help your body cope with medical treatments but it also helps you respond to the treatment better and encourages healing. Research has proven that chemotherapy works better when your pH levels are well balanced.

Can Help You Maintain a Healthy Weight

One of the major reasons why an alkaline-based diet has gained so much popularity is because it helps burn fat and bring you back in shape. Unlike other diet plans that promise you effective results in just 30 days, this diet plan helps you to stay fit and active and helps you to fight off diseases which are most important. When you shift from an acid-based diet to an alkaline diet, you automatically start lowering the amount of calories you consume and this helps your body burn fat faster. It also helps your body to get stronger and it gives you more energy.

Chapter 4 - Best Alkaline Foods

A common misconception about an alkaline based diet is that you need to simply shift to a vegan lifestyle and you start getting healthy. Although vegan food is good, in order for you to increase the alkalinity in your body, you have to consume foods that have high alkaline content.

Fresh Fruits And Vegetables

Following an effective alkaline diet entails including as much fruit and vegetable as possible. These fruits and vegetables work really well to balance the pH level in your body, making you healthier and more active. There is a variety you can purchase from the market but not all of these are great for alkaline diets. Here is a list of the most effective fruits and vegetables you should try to incorporate in your diet plan to increase alkaline levels in the body.

Avocado

Avocado is an amazing fruit when you are on an alkaline diet. Not only does it help reduce acidic levels in your body, but it also provides you with a lot of nutrients such as vitamin B, E, C and K. It also has a high content of potassium and copper along with monounsaturated healthy fats. Avocado contains dietary fiber which is great for your metabolism and also works well to aid weight loss because it helps you feel fuller for longer.

Broccoli

Although this vegetable isn't a favorite for a lot of people, including broccoli in your meals can give you a number of benefits. Broccoli is one of the few vegetables that are packed with nutrients that include Vitamin B6, K and C. It also has a high content of magnesium folate, Phosphorus Selenium and potassium that help diminish the acidic effects in your body and boost the alkaline content. It is always best to eat the vegetable raw.

Celery

Celery has high Vitamin B and C content. It also offers anti-inflammatory and antioxidant properties which help to enhance cardiovascular functionality. Celery helps to fight oxidative stress, keeping your body relieved and enhancing muscle mass as well as relaxing your muscles and your brain. Celery is a great vegetable to prevent dehydration since it has a lot of water content. The vegetable also has a lot of folate and potassium.

Cucumber

If there is one vegetable that can keep you hydrated all day long it's cucumber. Cucumber contains 96% water that helps increase your alkaline level and also releases your body of all the dirty toxins built up inside. Cucumbers are a rich source of vitamins and minerals such as Silicon, potassium and magnesium.

Lemon

Although a lot of people believe that lemon has high acidic content, the truth is it is actually alkaline that's inside the lemon. This citrus fruit works wonders on your digestive system and also help in better nutrition absorption. When making a salad, squeeze a generous amount of lemon on your meal and you will manage to absorb the nutrients in the salad a lot better. Vitamin C also helps to boost your immunity and protect your body against a number of illnesses because of the high Vitamin C content in it.

Peppers

Peppers are a great way to add flavor and color to your food. Whether you purchase green, yellow, or red bell peppers, they all have equal health benefits and provide you with a lot of Vitamin C and A. Peppers are also a great source of dietary fiber. Peppers contain a lot of antioxidants which help protect your body against cancer free radical cells.

Spinach

If Popeye taught you anything, it's to eat as much spinach as you can. This leafy vegetable has a high nutrient profile and it provides your body with vitamins A, C, B2 and K. It also contains high levels of iron, magnesium, manganese, folate, as well as iron. Another great benefit of eating spinach is that it helps improve the alkaline-acid ratio in your body.

All Raw Foods

The alkaline diet works best when you include raw food in your diet. The diet works well because you have kept the complete nutrition intact that the food has to offer. Whether it is in the shape of a salad, a soup or a smoothie, incorporate as much raw food as you can to boost your alkalinity and get healthier than ever before. One of the major reasons why you need to eat your food raw is because it's in the natural form and natural ingredients work best with alkalinity. When you cook your ingredients, it tends to lose a lot of the nutrients and it will not benefit your body as much as you would like it to. Some fruits and leafy vegetables have a high antioxidant content that are lost the minute it hits the heat. This is why you should try to incorporate as much raw food as possible in your diet. The best part about an alkaline diet is that you have a wide range of fruits and vegetables to choose from and these are best enjoyed raw.

Alkaline Water

When you adopt an alkaline diet, the one thing you need to learn is to prepare alkaline water. Alkaline water is nothing but water that has its alkaline levels boosted up to benefit you better. This water works wonders on your body and it helps to keep you healthy. One of the best things about alkaline water is that it has more hydrating properties in comparison to normal water, which means if you exercise or your body requires more water, the molecules in alkaline water can help rehydrate your body a lot faster than normal water.

Since the alkaline levels in the water are increased, it also boosts your immunity system and helps to fight off bacteria and infections more effectively. Regular consumption of alkaline water can work well to enhance your diet and take off all environmental toxins including stress. Unlike normal water, alkaline water contains a lot of magnesium and calcium and this contributes towards healthy bones. Since it has high antioxidant content, it also takes care of free radical cells and lowers the risk of cancer. Apart from fighting off diseases, alkaline water can also reverse the signs of aging and give you beautiful skin and hair. One of the best things about alkaline water is that it helps to lower the acidity in the system and it keeps your stomach and gastrointestinal tract healthy.

Green Drinks / Smoothies

Greens have become an integral part of your diet and they should be included in every form possible. While we have seen the benefits of including raw greens in your daily diet, including green drinks or green smoothies can also benefit your physical health in a number of ways. Here are a few benefits of green smoothies that you probably didn't know about.

Healthy Mentality

Green smoothies help you have a very positive and healthy frame of mind. The human mind is very difficult to train and it thrives on consistency. This means that if you start one particular habit that is healthy, your mind will start encouraging you to start another healthy habit. Try adding kale to your smoothie and see the mental change that it brings about. You will then want to take up a Yoga class that you have always wanted to try or go for a run on a daily basis when your smoothie intake is green.

Reduce Unhealthy Cravings

When you start consuming a green smoothie on a daily basis, you will feel nourished and not crave for unhealthy sweets or foods. This can again be tied to the mental frame of mind where your mind will want to continue the healthy transformation and encourage you to eat healthy snacks. Green smoothies are a great way to cut down on the binge eating and reduce the number of unhealthy snacks that you consume daily.

Glowing Skin

Since greens are rich in antioxidants, it does have a positive impact on your skin and you will see that your skin is hydrated and even the signs of aging have reduced.

Healthy Heart

As you are already aware, greens are rich in antioxidants and they help to lower your cholesterol and keep away heart-related problems.

Immunity Boost

Greens help boost your immune system and it will keep you away from illnesses for as long as you are consuming them. Consuming a green smoothie on a daily basis will keep you healthier than others who do not.

Better Digestion

Since smoothies utilize whole veggies, there is a lot of fiber that you receive and this will help improve your digestion.

Nutrient Absorption

When you consume smoothies daily, you will receive a lot of nutrients from vegetables such as spinach, kale, and lettuce.

Better Energy

When you start absorbing a lot of nutrients every day, your energy levels will be very high and you will feel very invigorated.

Other Foods

It's confusing to differentiate between foods that are highly acidic or alkaline, and that's the reason why people who just start out on an alkaline diet often end up eating the wrong kind of food. Just because something is vegan doesn't necessarily mean it is alkaline and it could benefit you. When you are on an alkaline diet, you should try and include alkaline fruits, nuts, legumes, and veggies. You should try to avoid foods that have high acid levels such as meat, poultry, fish, dairy, eggs, grains, and alcohol.

However, make sure that the fruits, nuts, legumes, and vegetables you include in your diet are highly alkaline and can promote the benefits of following the diet. There are some amazing alkaline foods that you should try to incorporate in your diet apart from the regular list that you will come across. These include soy products such as soya bean, miso, tofu, and tempeh. You can also look for unsweetened varieties of yogurt and curd as well as milk. Although some diets suggest that potatoes need to be avoided, you can most definitely include a small portion of potatoes when you are on an alkaline diet. You can also try to use as many herbs and spices to add flavor to your food.

Chapter 5 - Alkaline Herbs And Supplements

If you thought going on an alkaline diet means you need to avoid adding flavor to your food, then you couldn't be more wrong. As long as it"s healthy, you can use all kinds of spices and herbs to flavor your meal. The best part of an alkaline diet is you will find a wide range of herbs and supplements that you can use in your favor.

Herbs

Following an alkaline diet could get difficult because of the number of food items you need to stop consuming especially when you are used to being a non-vegetarian. However, when you look at the bright side of things, there are tons of herbs you can add to your meals to add flavor and make it more palatable. Here are some herbs that not only add flavor but also work wonders with your health.

Cayenne Pepper

Cayenne peppers add an amazing flavor to your food and while this is a pungent herb, it seems to be gaining a lot of popularity due to its taste. It has a lot of anti-inflammatory properties that work well to treat headaches and arthritis. It is also known to help reduce the signs of cancer. Cayenne pepper has also been associated with weight loss.

Dandelion Greens

Dandelion Greens can add amazing flavor to your salad and you can also use it to make herbal tea. It has high alkaline properties and is known to treat kidney stones effectively.

Turmeric

The bright yellow spice which is known to favor a number of curries has amazing properties and is also known to treat arthritis, cancer, and diabetes. It has a lot of medicinal properties and has been used by people for decades. If you can get your hands on fresh turmeric (the ones that look like ginger), you can use it not just to flavor your food but to make pickle and consume it with your meals. This works well to control your sugar levels and keep your bones healthy.

Garlic

The amazing antifungal and antibiotic properties that garlic has can help heal your body from within very effectively. Garlic is an amazing antioxidant and it also helps fight parasites in the body and making you stronger. Garlic is also known to be great for the heart and has high alkaline properties.

Supplements

Although there are a number of foods that can help increase the levels of alkaline in your body, sometimes you need a little assistance and in this situation, supplements play a vital role. Here are a few supplements that you may be advised to take depending on the kind of diet plan you follow.

Potassium Citrate and Magnesium Citrate

For alkalization to kick in, you need to have high levels of potassium and magnesium citrate. This is so that it lowers the amount of urine that is passed out of your body and also helps to enhance bone density and reduce the risk of brittle bones and fractures.

Calcium

Calcium is an important supplement that you may want to start consuming when on an alkaline diet not only because it keeps your bones healthy, but it also helps in reducing hypertension.

Glutamine

This supplement provides the body with amino acids which are necessary to lower the acidic levels and also helps to keep your kidney functioning effectively.

Vitamin D

Without adequate vitamin D in your body, it will not manage to absorb calcium and magnesium effectively. This is why it's also important you consume this supplement through the food you are eating.

Chapter 6 - Anti-Alkaline Foods And Habits

Starting off your alkaline diet might be tougher than you expected because of the various changes you need to make in your lifestyle in order to lower the acid levels and bring up your alkaline levels to an optimum level. There are various things that happen to your body when the acid levels are high and to bring this in control, it's necessary that you change your eating habits. The reason an alkaline diet is so necessary is because it helps reduce inflammation in the body which is one of the leading causes of various diseases including arthritis, diabetes, and cancer. It also causes chronic fatigue, irritability, unnecessary food cravings, and digestive problems. If you want to lead a healthy life and look great, it's important to address the root cause of all these problems which is high acid content in the body.

Once you bring your pH levels to the optimum level, it benefits you a great deal and you start feeling better about yourself. Not only do you manage to lose weight but you also feel more energetic and you drive away a number of illnesses. If you are diabetic, you will notice your sugar levels are in control and you will manage to get more done in a day because you simply feel great.

To follow a healthy alkaline diet, make sure you avoid meat and fish, food that contains any dairy product, eggs, alcohol, or nicotine and drugs, as well as refined grains of processed food. You should also try and stay away from any food items that have high sugar content as this isn't good for your body. Packaged cereal is also something you may want to avoid along with fast food. These foods have high acid levels and are not recommended during an alkaline diet.

Although alkaline diets do not recommend it, you avoid roasted nuts and seeds, tofu, tempeh, and soya bean in any form. It is highly recommended that you control eating these food items and never eat them more than twice a week. Food items that include vinegar or apple cider can be included in your diet more often since it's high alkaline. Avoid processed chocolates and dry fruits which have sugar added to it. Readymade salad dressings should also be limited since they are not great to consume on a daily basis.

If you want to train your mind to eat healthily, you need to take small steps and start with a few changes at a time so that your body gets used to it. If you are a hardcore non-vegetarian and you eat meats 5 to 6 times a week, do not give it up completely but instead decrease the size and limit your intake until you are comfortable giving it up and following an alkaline diet. An important rule to follow when choosing a diet plan, irrespective of which one it is, is to not force your body and make sure that whatever you plan on doing, your body is fine with it.

High-Sodium Foods: Processed Foods

Processed foods are unhealthy, which is why they should be avoided completely whether or not you are on an alkaline diet. One of the major reasons why they are so bad is because most processed foods are loaded with sugar that adds unnecessary calories in your body and doesn't benefit you in any way. Processed foods contain no fiber content which means they affect your digestion and they don't work well for your metabolism levels as well. Processed foods are highly addictive and this means that once you get hooked on to eating these foods, it is going to be difficult for you to stop. They are known to cause mood swings and they can lead to irritability and sometimes put you in a depressed state of mind. Most processed foods have high sodium content that is not healthy for you and is known to increase blood pressure. Processed food also interferes with your sleeping habits, making it difficult for you to get sound sleep. Since these food items are made to last long, they are loaded with preservatives which could take a longer time to digest and eventually lead to a lot of weight gain.

Cold Cuts And Conventional Meats

When you lead a hectic life, cold cuts could work as a savior as they are just sitting in the freezer waiting for you to pull out and make a sandwich or a quick meal out of it. What most people don't realize is cold cuts are generally the main cause of health-related problems including high blood pressure, obesity, and high cholesterol. Cold cuts are cured meats which are preserved either by salting or smoking, and in some cases are preserved with chemicals such as sodium nitrate, all of which have high health risks. They have a lot of unnecessary calories and should be avoided if you want to lead a healthy life. Reducing the amount of cold cuts in your diet can help reduce the risk of cancer, according to the World Health Organisation.

Processed Cereals

Processed cereals are easy to use for people who are always on the rush. The problem with processed cereal is that it either has a lot of sugar content or the ones that are low on sugar levels contain artificial sweeteners, both of which are highly acidic for the body. These contain toxic ingredients that only destroy your body over time and don't benefit you in any way. They do not have any nutrients and only keep you full for a couple of hours before your body starts craving for more junk food.

Eggs

Eggs are a controversial subject when it comes to following an alkaline diet because an alkaline diet asks you to avoid it completely. While they usually say that an egg is healthy, the truth is consuming it may not be as beneficial as you imagine them to be. While they are high in protein content, eggs also contain a lot of cholesterol which is not great for your system and can increase the risk of a heart attack and clogged arteries. High cholesterol levels are often linked with liver cancer which is why you may want to avoid eating an egg if you want to keep your liver healthy. It is also believed that eggs contain chlorine, a compound that is highly toxic and starts growing in the gut of the person thereby increasing the risk of various health conditions. Eggs are also known to be highly acidic which affects the alkaline levels in your body and causes multiple health issues.

Caffeinated Drinks and Alcohol

Drinks that have high caffeine form bubbles in the stomach causing it to expand and giving you the feeling of bloatedness. This is an uncomfortable feeling not only because you start feeling sick, but also because it affects your digestive system. Foods that contain caffeine and aerated drinks are highly acidic and should be avoided when you are on an alkaline diet and trying to get healthy. These drinks are also often loaded with a lot of sugar which adds unnecessary calories to your diet.

When you start an alkaline diet, the first thing you need to get out of your list is alcohol because alcohol is highly acidic and it could increase the amount of gastric acid in your system. The worst part about alcohol is people start consuming it with a number of carbonated drinks that multiplies the problem and creates uncomfortable situations for your body. Alcohol is not good for your liver and people who drink are more prone to liver-related issues including enlargement of the liver and cirrhosis of the liver, both of which can be avoided by cutting down on your alcohol consumption. Let's not forget, alcohol and caffeine interfere with your pH balance and push you more towards the acidic side.

Oats and Whole Wheat Products

Oats and whole wheat may sound amazing to consume when you are on a diet but these are also food products you may want to avoid when you switch to an alkaline diet. Although oats and whole wheat are healthy, the problem with both these items is that they are complex carbohydrates that take a longer time to break down in your body, thereby making it difficult for the body to digest the food. This increases the acid levels in your system and makes it difficult to maintain a healthy pH balance when you are trying to get your body"s alkaline levels high.

Milk

As a child, you were told you should drink a glass of milk to make your bones healthy. The truth however, is that cow"s milk actually takes off the Calcium from your bones. While calcium is an amazing acid neutralizer, milk isn't and it tends to add more acid to your body than you can imagine. This means every time you drink a glass of milk, your body is drained of the calcium content thereby increasing the acid levels.

Several researchers have proven that milk can lead to prostate cancer which is why people should switch to soy milk instead. Your body needs a lot of time to digest milk and if it isn't digested properly, it could lead to bloating, diarrhea, and cramps that could make you uncomfortable.

Milk also has a lot of cholesterol, and regular consumption can increase your cholesterol levels quite a bit. Research has proven that people who consume more milk are more prone to ovarian cancer. If you have heard that you should only use antibiotics when prescribed by a doctor and always complete the dosage so that your body does not start building a resistance towards the medication, you may want to stay off milk because cow"s milk contains antibiotics and they start entering your system the minute you drink it and creates an anti drug-resistant atmosphere in your body. You won't even know what drugs you are resistant to because you haven't consumed them directly. Milk is often linked to weight gain and people who drink milk on a regular basis tend to add more weight in comparison to those who don't. You can substitute milk with soy-based milk products that are healthy and more alkaline in nature.

Peanuts and Walnuts

While an alkaline diet asks you to consume nuts on a regular basis, you need to stay away from peanuts and walnuts for a reason. Both peanuts and walnuts are known to increase the acid levels in your body and this is why you may want to stay away from them. These nuts interfere with the pH balance in your body and make it difficult for you to come to the level of alkalinity that you wish. These nuts are also known to create multiple health issues including congestion and interference in the detoxification process during an alkaline diet. Unlike most of the other nuts that help you to lose weight, peanuts and walnuts are generally associated with weight gain which is why you may want to stay away from them during your alkaline diet.

Pasta, Rice, Bread and Packaged Grain Products

If you are starting an alkaline diet, the one thing you have to lay off is your pasta, rice, and bread for a reason. They are known to cause the number of dietary issues because of the heavy carbohydrates and starch content that they have. These increase the acidity in your body and are known to cause gas and heat burn along with bloating. They are also known to release complex sugars which are difficult to digest and gets accumulated as fat in your body.

The Kind Of Habits That Can Cause Acidity In Your Body

If you are going on an alkaline diet, it isn't just about what you eat but also what you need to avoid to get healthy. If you want your alkaline diet to go well, you need to identify the biggest offender of the diet and stay as far away from them as possible.

Alcohol and Drugs

We have already understood that alcohol has high acid content which is why you should avoid it. Alcohol has many underlying effects as well such as causing depression and stress on a person. The problem with alcohol is that it's addictive and just like drugs, it could make you lethargic and lazy. Drugs are also high in acid content and when you start consuming drugs or start smoking on a regular basis, you are increasing the acid content in your body. If you want to follow a healthy alkaline diet, you need to cut off the alcohol and stop smoking or stop consuming drugs in any form.

High Caffeine Intake

Caffeine in any form should be avoided because it interferes with the functionality of your body and increases your heart rate unnecessarily. Caffeine also has high acid content along with a lot of unwanted sugar which results in weight gain. Consuming too many caffeine products will interfere with your sleeping habit and this causes stress as well as improper functionality of the organs.

Antibiotic Overuse

When you start popping pills unnecessarily, this does not benefit you in any way and it makes your body so used to those medicines that they won't work even when you actually have an infection that needs to be treated. These infections are known as drug-resistant infections and they are only caused when you abuse antibiotics and consume them over your recommended amount. Too much antibiotics also result in acid reflux and high acidity levels in your body which has a number of side effects and affects your alkaline diet.

Artificial Sweeteners

Artificial sweeteners are highly acidic and interfere with the process of an alkaline diet. If you want to stay healthy, you have to learn to avoid your cravings for sweets and this includes artificial sweeteners. The best artificial sweeteners are registered as low as 2.5 on a pH balance scale meaning that they are extremely acidic. If you continue using artificial sweeteners in your diet, you will not manage to bring your pH balance to the alkaline level you desire and the diet will not work as planned.

Chronic Stress

High stress level usually results in acidity and acid reflux, which is why it's important for you to learn how to relax and calm your body before you take on an alkaline diet. If you suffer from serious stress, it is going to be very difficult for you to control your acid levels in the body and this could mean that following the diet may not benefit you in the way you want, no matter how many alkalizing foods you consume. If you are going through too much stress, the best thing to do would be to consult a doctor and bring your stress levels in control before you start the diet plan.

To get the best out of your alkaline diet, it's important that you learn how to identify acidic food items and stay away from them. Apart from that, here are some basic tips you may want to follow in order to make the most out of the alkaline diet plan and lead a healthy life.

Eat Regularly

It is important for you to make time to eat regular and healthy meals if you want your body to get into control. No matter how busy you are, try to make time to ensure you eat the right amount of food multiple times a day rather than stuffing too much food two or three times a day.

Sleep Well

If you want to get healthy and want the alkaline diet to work, you need to provide your body with enough rest every day. You should try and get at least seven to eight hours of sleep because this helps relax your body and also relieves your body from a lot of acids, making you feel unhealthy.

Stop Smoking

If you want the alkaline diet to work, you need to say goodbye to your smoking habit so that it benefits you and you manage to make the diet a successful one. This will not only help you in weight loss but will also drive away diseases and increase your energy levels.

Low Levels of Nutrients in Foods Due to Industrial Farming

When you start to follow an alkaline diet, the one thing you may want to focus on is purchasing products that are organic and homegrown. Products that are available on an industrial level do not contain the number of nutrients as you would want them to because they are mass produced and usually chemical based. Thankfully, there are farmers markets that are available in every locality and if there is one close to you, make the most of it and purchase all fresh fruits and vegetables from a farmers market so that you get homegrown and organic food products.

Low Levels of Fiber in the Diet

When you follow an alkaline diet, the one thing you need to make sure is that you provide your body with enough fiber so that it functions effectively and you manage to eliminate the dirty toxins that you are suffering from. If you want to lose weight during the alkaline diet, fiber plays an essential role in easing better digestion. Broccoli, apples, and carrots are high in fiber so when you start your diet, make sure to include plenty of these on a daily basis.

Including Non Grass-Fed Animal Meats in the Diet

It is not easy for a non-vegetarian to switch to an alkaline diet that is completely vegan, and this is why you may want to cut down the amount of meat you include in your daily life without completely eliminating it. However, there are meats that are non grass-fed that you may want to try and avoid because these are higher in fat and calories. Grass-fed meat manages to provide you with proteins which benefit you. While your goal should be to give up on meat completely, you can always start by reducing the amount of meat you eat and choosing a flexitarian diet for a few days.

Eliminating Unnecessary Hormones from Your Life

In order for you to stay healthy, it is important to identify your exposure to hidden hormones. These hormones could be found in a variety of food items and beauty products as well as plastics that you are often exposed to. The best way to understand where the hidden hormones lie is to check for the level of chemicals in the product because that's what usually relates to as a hidden hormone. If you want to lower the risk of exposure to these hidden hormones, you might want to try opting in for natural products, whether it's for food or your beauty products or even plastic and try to limit the amount of chemicals in your life.

Radiation

Electromagnetic radiation can cause a number of side effects in your life and while we believe we keep ourselves away from this exposure, the truth is there are a number of products you use on a daily basis including your cell phone and your microwave that release this radiation more than you would like them to. If you want to stay healthy, you should try to stop heating food in a microwave and make smaller portions that you finish up in one consumption. You should also sleep away from your cell phone so that it does not affect you while you sleep.

Preservatives in Food Coloring

While natural food coloring is still manageable, artificial food colors are full of chemicals and preservatives which do not work well on your body and may slow down the process of digestion. This also affects your vital organs which is why you should stay away from any product that has preservatives or artificial food coloring.

Pesticides

Pesticides are harmful to the environment and while a lot of people know this, what they don't realize is these pesticides can also be extremely harmful to the human body as well. Prolonged exposure to pesticides can lead to various health-related issues and can increase the risk of cancer. If you believe organic is something that is just a little more expensive, then you may want to reconsider because too much of pesticides could increase neurological disorders such as Parkinson's disease, leukemia, asthma, and other diseases in your body. An alkaline diet always recommends raw, organic and natural foods as a force to the ones that are treated with pesticides for the obvious reasons.

Over-Exercise

It's common for people to feel pumped once they start any diet plan and they always like to accompany it with an exercise regime. While exercise is great, it's important for you to make sure you don't overdo it because an excess of anything will be bad and that is also true for exercise. If you attempt exercising more than your body can handle, you could end up with a muscle tear or tissue damage that could take months to heal. Instead of doing too much on one day, you may want to start slow but make sure that you don't miss a single day of exercise so that your body gets movement regularly and you manage to burn fat and increase your energy levels effectively.

Pollution

Although it is hard to stay away from pollution, this is something that could affect your body in various ways on a regular basis. High pollution levels can cause damage to your lungs, brain, and heart. The reason why an alkaline diet is recommended is because this helps clean your organs and increases the strength of your lungs as well as cleanses your heart and removes all the dirty toxins and pollutants from your body regularly.

Poor Chewing and Eating Habits

One of the worst things that you can do is to eat your food too quickly. The faster you swallow, the higher the chances of you staying overweight because it takes a while for bigger food particles to digest in the body as compared to smaller particles that you chew properly. It is also said that you should eat your food slower because this gives your body enough time to digest the food more effectively and drinking water in between your meals definitely helps you to stay fitter in comparison to those who start chewing and swallowing the food really fast.

Shallow Breathing

Most people lead a hectic life and they literally have no time to take a deep breath! If you want to stay healthy, it's important to breathe easily and with comfort rather than taking short breaths and trying to take in as much air in a short shallow breath as possible. The deeper your breaths are, the more relaxed your body is and the better it is for your lungs. In case you have a breathing problem and you are used to taking shorter breaths, you may want to start practicing taking deep breaths at least five to six times a day until you get into the habit of it.

Chapter 7: Dr Sebi's 10 Day Cleanse

Dr. Sebi had introduced a 10 day cleanse that helps you eat healthy while keeping up with the demands of a busy lifestyle. There are a number of foods that are available on the go, however these foods will make your body very unhealthy and you will be filled with a lot of negative sensations. These foods such as red meat, fast food, and greasy foods lead to a lot of weight gain as well as health complications and heart problems.

Over a period of time, you will realize that your energy is considerably low and this is something that can be avoided with the help of Dr. Sebi"s 10 day cleanse. If you are already too far ahead in terms of eating unhealthy foods and are not feeling great about your weight that you have put on, you may want to try this 10 day cleanse and it will help bring your body back on track. This 10 day cleanse helps to remove all the low energy from your body and it will also relieve you of the stress that you are going through.

Understanding The 10 Day Cleanse

Following the 10 day cleanse is not as easy as it sounds and you need a lot of discipline in order to make sure that you get your body's balance back in place. The key to the 10 day cleanse is to make sure that you keep away from all kinds of acidic foods and you drink natural spring water. There are four different ways that you can go about doing the Dr. Sebi 10 day cleanse. Here is what each of them comprises of.

Fasting

One of the hardest ways to go about Dr. Sebi"s 10 day cleanse is with fasting. While fasting may seem difficult, it is definitely the most effective when it comes to reversing various health conditions that you are undergoing. Before you try the option of fasting, you need to make sure that you consult your doctor and see if you are fit enough to go through with this process. The fasting process mainly focuses on eating sea moss and drinking spring water. Your food intake is severely limited during this cleansing process and it may be difficult to sustain it if your body is not strong enough.

Juice Cleanse

As the name states, this is a juice cleansing process and you are able to consume all kinds of fruits and vegetables in their liquid form. If you feel that only juices may not keep you going, then you may want to add a bit of sea moss powder or sea moss gel after drinking your juice. This will ensure that you do not give in to your hunger temptations and you stay on track with the cleansing process. Before you go ahead with this cleansing process, you need to make sure that you invest in a blender that is very reliable as well as stable.

Food and Juice Cleanse

This is definitely one of the best cleansers to make sure that you stay on track with the cleansing process and you achieve your weight loss goals. This cleanse recommends that you eat raw foods as much as possible; however if you are not able to do that, you should stick to the recommended foods by Dr. Sebi. The first few days of this cleanse are very difficult however, if you make it past the first four days, you will be able to complete the 10 days successfully. The best part about this cleanse is that you will not crave for any kind of junk food after just one week.

Food, Juice as well as Herb Cleanse

Adding herbs to your cleansing process can definitely help make the cleanse more effective. The reason a lot of people add herbs to their cleanse is it helps to remove all the toxins from the body and it will also improve the mindset of the person. The people that are on this cleanse can consume vegetable broth as well as all kinds of fruits and vegetable juices. You can even eat vegetables, fruits, nuts, salads, as well as grains. You need to make sure that everything you consume is fresh and natural as this will help to reset the balance of your body and remove all the toxins successfully.

Enhancing The 10 Day Cleanse

While the 10 day cleanse is not very easy, you can enhance the cleanse further by adding herbs to it. Irrespective of the kind of cleanse you are doing, you can add herbs to your diet and this will take your cleanse to the next level. You can purchase herbal supplements that are available in capsule form and this will help you go through the day without having the need to rely on solid foods. A number of people that are on liquid cleanses often give up after the second day because they are not able to stay away from solid foods. These herbal supplements will help your body feel good and it will also help Dr. Sebi‟s cleansing process to be successful.

Conclusion

With so many diet plans being introduced into the market on a regular basis, it is natural to get confused with regards to which one will work and which ones make absolutely no sense! If you are looking to lose weight without staying concerned about your health, then you should probably look for something that works fast and has no logic to it. While these kinds of diet plans often attract more customers, they are the kind of diet plans that eventually fail because they don't live up to their expectations and once somebody gives up the diet, they get back to the way they were or even heavier.

The reason an alkaline diet is so perfectly crafted is because it doesn't just focus on losing weight, but it also includes crucial steps that help reduce and reverse the risks of life-threatening diseases including cancer and diabetes. An alkaline diet is the only diet that can help cure you from within and you will feel better and more energetic in no time.

An alkaline diet may be difficult to start off with but once you start it, you will realize how amazing you feel and you'll never want to get off this diet plan in your life. One small step towards a healthy future can pave the path for a happy, stress-free, younger, energetic and beautiful you! Take that step today and adapt to an alkaline way of life!

One Meal a Day Intermittent Fasting

*Guide to Losing Fat,
Increasing your Spirituality
and Getting More Work Done*

J.P. Edwin

advice. The content of this book has been derived from various sources. Please consult a licensed professional before attempting any techniques outlined in this book.

By reading this document, the reader agrees that under no circumstances is the author responsible for any losses, direct or indirect, which are incurred as a result of the use of information contained within this document, including, but not limited to, —errors, omissions, or inaccuracies.

Introduction

I want to thank you for choosing this book, „*One Meal a Day Intermittent Fasting - Guide to Losing Fat, Increasing your Spirituality and Getting More Work Done.*"

Are you looking for a diet that will help you lose weight and improve your health? Do you want a diet that doesn"t insist on counting calories? Imagine if you could achieve your fitness and weight loss goals without counting calories! That does sound quite wonderful, doesn"t it? If your answer is yes, then intermittent fasting is the diet that you were searching for.

The concept of fasting is not a new one and it has been around since time immemorial. People tend to fast for medical, health or even spiritual reasons. Intermittent fasting is a simple dieting protocol that alternates between periods of fasting and eating.

In this book, you will learn about the One Meal a Day protocol of intermittent fasting. You will also read about the basics of intermittent fasting, the changes that take place in your body while fasting, different methods of intermittent fasting, the benefits it offers, tips for weight loss and the spirituality of fasting. Apart from this, you will also learn about the different ways in which this diet improves your overall productivity so that you can get more Work done! Also, the success stories given in this book will inspire you to try this diet for yourself.

So, if you are ready to learn more about this wonderful diet that can turn your life around, then let us get started right away!

Chapter One: What is OMAD and Intermittent Fasting?

Intermittent fasting is a simple concept - you are free to eat almost anything that you want for a specific period of time and then you need to fast for a while until it is time to eat again. During the fasting period, you are free to eat anything that doesn"t have any calories in it. Intermittent fasting is a simple concept and you can find a method that will suit your personal needs.

Unlike other forms of traditional dieting, the idea of fasting is quite unambiguous and easy to understand. Did you know that most of us tend to fast from time to time anyway? Usually, we tend to fast without thinking about it, and it isn"t a conscious decision. When you think about it, did you ever skip a meal in a day? If you did, then you were following an intermittent fasting protocol. You will learn about the different methods of intermittent fasting in the coming chapters.

Our caveman ancestors were predominantly hunters and gatherers. So, if they needed to eat, they had to hunt or search for food in nature. It meant that they used to fast until they found some form of nourishment. Then agriculture came along, and it led to the creation of human civilization. Whenever there was scarcity of food or whenever the seasons changed, fasting was the norm of life. It was a common practice to maintain stores of grain and meat in the cities and castles to survive harsh winters. Before the advent of agriculture, a shortage of rainfall meant a spell of famine and people used to fast to ensure that their food supplies would last them longer. Sufficient rain was a precondition to meet the necessary grain requirement.

Religions cropped up with the civilizations. Religions grew when people started to live in close quarters and started to share similar beliefs. Most of these religions tended to prescribe some form of fasting. In Hinduism, fasting is known as Vaasa and is said to be a form of penance. Islam prescribes fasting during the holy month of Ramadan. A similar practice exists in Judaism and is known as Yom Kippur. Even Christianity prescribes fasting before Easter.

Technology and innovation played a major role in the evolution of human beings. Industrialization completely revolutionized the food industry. It introduced the concept of mass production of food products. It meant that the markets are flooded with food products all the time. Apart from this, the way human beings view and consume food has also undergone a massive overhaul. The world that humans live in has changed a lot, but the human body didn't get an opportunity to acclimatize itself to the changes that were brought about by industrialization and the advent of agriculture. All this does signify the growth of the human race, but it also meant the introduction of a variety of health problems that humans were not used to. The practice of intermittent fasting can be traced back centuries. Even though it is an old practice, humans have just started to fully understand and appreciate the different benefits this diet provides. Whenever you are fasting, you tend to give your body a chance to cleanse itself from within. Not just cleanse, but even regenerate and repair itself from within.

While you are fasting, your body gets an opportunity to burn all the excess fat that it keeps stored within. Humans have evolved in such a manner that it is quite safe to fast, and there are no risks involved in fasting. The body fat stored in the cells is the reserve of food that the body stores away for a rainy day. When you don"t consume any food, your body merely reaches into its internal stores to provide energy.

It is the law of nature that there needs to be balance in all aspects of life. The Chinese concept of yin and yang is quite practical and these rules apply to eating and fasting too. Eating and fasting are the two sides of a single coin. Fasting is the flipside of eating so when you don't eat, you are fasting. Whenever you eat something, it leads to the accumulation of energy that your body doesn't use immediately. A portion of all that you eat is stored away for later use. Insulin, a hormone that is secreted by pancreas is responsible for storing energy. Whenever you eat something, there is a spike of insulin in your body. Insulin helps the body store energy in two different ways. The sugars are linked into long chains known as glycogen and the rest is stored in the liver.

There is only so much fat that the liver can hold onto so, the rest is sent to different cells in the body in the form of fat. Liver stores some fat and the rest is safely stowed away in different cells. There is no limit to the amount of fat that the body can churn out. There are two forms of energy that are present in the body. One of these forms is easily accessible but has a limited storage space and is known as glycogen. The other form of energy is harder to reach into and has an unlimited storage space, which is known as body fat.

When you don"t eat anything, your body reverses this process. There will be a decline in the level of insulin and it encourages your body to dip into its stores of fat. Once your body accesses this fat, it starts to burn it to provide energy. Glycogen is the most easily attainable source of energy in the body. It is quite easy to break the glycogen molecules down to provide energy. The energy that"s produced like this can sustain your body for 24 hours or even longer. After your body exhausts its reserves of glucose, it starts to burn fat to provide energy.

Your body will continue to do this only when you are eating or fasting. Either your body is burning energy or it is storing energy. Only one of these processes can take place at a time. If there is a balance between when you eat and fast, then it doesn"t lead to any weight gain. Over a period, you will start to put on weight if you don"t give your body the time it needs to burn the food that it is storing within. To restore the quintessential balance in your body, you need to give it plenty of time to burn the stored food for energy. If you want to accomplish this, then intermittent fasting is necessary. In fact, this is precisely how our bodies are designed by nature. Intermittent fasting helps restore this balance.

Circadian Rhythm and Intermittent Fasting

Like all the other organisms on this Earth, even human beings have an internal circadian clock that ensures that all the physiological processes are being performed at the right time. The circadian rhythm is switched on all day long and it has an effect on the biology as well as the behavior of human beings.

Any disruption in the circadian rhythm will have a negative effect on the metabolism and it causes various metabolic dysfunctions like obesity, diabetes and a host of cardiovascular problems. The primary factor that regulates the circadian rhythm is the signal to feed. It is responsible for the functioning of all the metabolic, physiological and behavioral pathways in the body. In turn, all these different pathways are responsible to ensure that your body performs optimally. Apart from this, the circadian rhythm also ensures that your body is healthy. A form of behavioral intervention is necessary to regulate the circadian rhythm in the body. Yes, you guessed it right! The behavioral intervention that I am talking about is intermittent fasting. Intermittent fasting helps streamline the circadian rhythm. All this helps to improve the gene expression and leads to an overall improvement in your body"s health as well as metabolism.

Gut Microbiome and Intermittent Fasting

The gastrointestinal tract is responsible for regulating various processes within your body. In other words, your gut is responsible for regulating various physiological and biochemical functions going on in your body. For instance, did you know that the metabolic reaction to glucose as well as blood flow tend to be higher during the day than at night? Even a slight fluctuation in the circadian rhythm tends to impair your metabolism and it increases the risk factor of different chronic health problems. The microbiome that"s present in the gut is known as the second brain. It is referred to as such because it exerts certain control over your overall metabolism and physiology. Intermittent fasting tends to have a positive effect on the gut microbiome. It tends to make the gut less permeable, reduces the chances of systemic inflammation and improves the balance of energy.

Lifestyle Behavior and Intermittent Fasting

Intermittent fasting also helps change different behaviors important for health like the sleep cycle, calorie consumption and energy usage. Therefore, it doesn"t come as a surprise that any imbalance in these three is the primary reason for any health concern. You will learn more about the different benefits of intermittent fasting in the coming chapters.

Different Methods of Fasting

16/8 method

The 16/8 method is one of the easiest intermittent fasting protocols there is. We are all effectively fasting while asleep and this method is simply an extension of that fasting period. Most of us tend to skip our breakfast and tend to have our first meal after 12 noon. Well, in this method of fasting, you simply have to make sure that your eating window doesn"t exceed 8 hours. In this process, an individual is required to fast for 16 hours in a day. The eating window is restricted to 8 hours. Two regular or three small meals can be squeezed into this period. This method is quite simple to follow. It can be something as simple as skipping breakfast or not munching on anything after dinner. For instance, you can make sure that the last meal that you have is at 8 in the evening. Make sure that you don"t eat anything until 12 noon the following day. It provides you with a fasting window of about 16 hours. It has been observed that it would be better if women fast for a shorter duration of time and don"t let their fasting period go beyond 14-15 hours. For those who feel hungry in the morning and are used to having breakfast every day, this can be hard initially. However, if you were already used to skipping breakfast, then it will be easy. You can have water, coffee and other beverages that don"t have many calories in them while you are fasting. If you are just getting started with intermittent fasting, then this is the fasting protocol that you must consider.

5:2 Diet

If the idea of fasting daily doesn"t appeal to you, then you can follow the 5:2 dieting protocol. While following this diet, the individual gets to eat regularly on five days of the week and restricts the calorie intake to 500-600 calories on the other two days of the week. This diet is referred to as the Fast diet. On the two fasting days, it is recommended that women must have 500 calories and men can consume 600 calories. For instance, you get to eat regularly on all days except the two days when you want to fast. On such days, you can eat two meals consisting of 250-300 calories each depending on your gender. This diet is suitable for all those who feel that they cannot fast for the whole day and who would like to eat a little something. 5:2 diet is a very simple diet. You have control over deciding the days on which you want to fast and the days on which you don"t. If you don"t like the idea of abstaining from eating, then this is well suited for you. The days when you are fasting, you can either stick to a strict diet or give yourself permission to have around 500 calories.

Eat-stop-Eat

This form of intermittent fasting requires the individual to fast for 24 hours, once or twice every week. You will need to fast for 24 hours consecutively on this diet. From dinner on one day until dinner the consecutive day, that will constitute 24 hours. For instance, you had your dinner at 7 p.m. on Monday, and you don"t get to eat until 7 p.m. on Tuesday. This will be the 24 hours fasting window. You can also do this from breakfast on a given day until breakfast on the following day. You will just need to fast for 24 hours; you can select the timings according to your convenience. You cannot consume any solid food during this diet. However, water, coffee and other beverages that don‟t have any calories in them can be safely consumed. If you are following this method because you want to lose weight, then in such a case you will need to eat regularly during your feeding window. You must eat the sort of food you are used to eating, had you not been fasting. The only problem with this method is that there happens to be a 24-hour fasting window and it might be difficult for a few people to follow. You don‟t have to start out with this necessarily. You can gradually progress from the 16-hour fasting model. The first stretch of the diet will not be hard; it is only toward the end that this diet gets a little complicated to follow. This is where discipline and motivation will come in handy.

If you keep yourself busy, then you won‟t have time to think about food or hunger. So, on the fasting days, make sure that you keep yourself busy or engaged. Plan your day so that you are indulging in activities that keep you occupied. You must have plenty of water. Not only will it keep your body thoroughly hydrated, but it will also leave you feeling full for longer. Make sure that you plan your week in such a manner that your fasting days don‟t clash with any other social obligations. Intermittent fasting protocols are quite convenient, and you don't have to compromise on your social life for the sake of this diet.

Alternate day fasting

As the name suggests, this diet is all about fasting on every alternate day. There are different variations of this diet. If you want, you can fast for 24-hours on every alternate day and then there are other variations that allow you to eat about 500 calories on every alternate day, and the others require you to observe a strict fast on every alternate day. Most of the lab studies that have been conducted to find the benefits of intermittent fasting have made use of some variation of this diet. A strict fast might sound rather severe and extreme. Depending upon your comfort level, you can adapt this diet to suit your needs. It is advisable that beginners don't immediately jump to this method. With this method of fasting, be prepared to go to bed hungry a few times every week. This diet doesn't show any form of sustainability in the long run.

Warrior diet

This kind of fasting involves the consumption of small quantities of raw fruit and veggies during the day and then consuming a single hearty meal at night. Mostly, you will need to fast throughout the day, and then you get to feast at night. The feeding window extends to only 4 hours. This variation of the intermittent fasting diets was one of the first ones to be popular. While following this method of fasting, the food choices that you make must be quite similar to what you will have made had you been following the Paleo diet. You will need to consume foods that are unprocessed. You can eat anything that our cavemen ancestors will have consumed. If something looks like it was produced in a factory, you must certainly avoid it.

The Paleo diet is a high fat and a low carb diet, just like the ketogenic diet. The protocols of a Paleo diet can be successfully combined with the dieting protocols of an intermittent fast. For instance, if you are following the alternate day model of fasting, then on the days when you aren"t fasting you must follow a Paleo diet. You just have to make sure that whenever you are eating, the food that you are consuming is Paleo-friendly. So, you cannot have any form of processed foods, starchy foods or carbs. By combining these two diets, you can reap the benefits of the Paleo diet and intermittent fasting as well.

Skipping meals spontaneously

Well, this is an obvious one and this form of intermittent fasting doesn"t have a structured plan. You will simply have to skip meals spontaneously from time to time. Skip meals whenever you aren"t hungry, or you are preoccupied with some work. If you aren"t hungry, then don"t eat. It is as simple as that. Just skip a meal whenever you feel like it. Then depending on how hungry you are you can have a hearty meal after that. However, you will need to make sure that the other meals that you are consuming are healthy. Skipping meals is not the same as starvation. Don"t try to starve yourself, that"s not what this method is about. By skipping meals when you aren"t hungry, you are reducing the unnecessary calorie consumption. Your body knows what it needs and learn to listen to it. Eat only when you are hungry.

One Meal a Day Diet

The popularity of intermittent fasting is increasing every day. One method of IF that is steadily becoming quite popular is the One Meal a Day diet also known as the OMAD diet. Abstaining from food helps modulate your body"s performance and when you fast for prolonged periods, it has a positive effect on your body and mind.

The OMAD protocol is designed in such a manner that the fasting ratio you need to follow is 23:1. It means that your body will be effectively fasting for 23 hours and the eating window is restricted to one hour. If you want to burn fat, trigger weight loss, improve your mental clarity and reduce the time that you spend on food, then eating one meal a day is a brilliant idea.

The OMAD method oscillates between periods of eating and fasting. This method of fasting reduces the eating window more than the other diets. While following this dieting protocol, you need to make sure that you consume your daily calories within one meal and you fast for the rest of the day. OMAD helps you reap all the benefits of intermittent fasting and it simplifies your schedule as well. The ideal time to break your fast is between 4 and 7 p.m. When you do this, you give your body sufficient time to start digesting the food that you eat before you sleep.

From the perspective of evolution, humans aren"t designed to eat three meals per day. As mentioned earlier, our ancestor"s bodies were used to functioning optimally even when there was food scarcity. Intermittent fasting protocols like the OMAD tend to kickstart various cell functions in your body that are helpful to improve your overall health. It can be quite intimidating to get started with this method of dieting. There are three simple tips that you can follow to make the transition easier on yourself.

The first thing that you need to do is **slowly cut back on the carbs** that you consume. If you want to optimize the results of this diet and want the least amount of crankiness, then you must limit your carb intake. When you consume a lot of carbs, your body tends to create a stock of glycogen in the body. If there is always some glucose present in your body, then your body will not be able to shift into ketosis. Ketosis is essential to kickstart the process of burning fats. So, if you are trying to start this diet, then it is a good idea to start by slowly cutting back on your carb intake.

You need to **ease your body into getting used to this fasting protocol**. It can be quite difficult to go from eating three meals a day to just one meal a day. You need to ease the transition so that it doesn"t feel like you are suffering. A simple way in which you can do this is by slowly getting your body used to the idea of eating fewer meals. So, if you are used to eating three meals per day and tend to snack in between the meals, then the first step is to eliminate all the snacks. Then you can slowly increase the time between the meals and cut down on the number of meals you eat. If you do this, it will be quite easy to follow this diet.

Another simple way in which you can make this diet easier on your body is to consume some caffeine. A morning cup of coffee (devoid of milk and sugar) will make you feel fuller for longer and will keep your hunger pangs at bay. You will learn more about the different tips that you can follow to manage your hunger in the coming chapters.

Chapter Two: Weight Loss

Your body tends to store energy in the form of fat cells. When you don"t eat anything, there a couple of different changes that take place in your body that help your body access its energy reserves. There are a couple of changes that take place in the activity of your nervous system. Here are a couple of changes that take place in the metabolism of your body whenever you fast.

Insulin- The level of insulin increases whenever you eat. So, while you are fasting, the insulin levels in your body will decrease. A low level of insulin means that it is easier for your body to burn the fats that are stored within.

Human Growth Hormone - The human growth hormone or HGH level increases when you fast. This hormone is responsible for not just fat loss, but it also helps with muscle gain and it kick starts autophagy.

Noradrenaline - Norepinephrine or noradrenaline is sent to the fat cells by the nervous system to help break down the fat in the body and to free up the reserves of fatty acids to provide energy.

If you keep consuming food throughout the day, then it is unlikely that any of these changes will take place. Short-term fasting helps increase your body"s ability to burn fats. So, a short-term fast like intermittent fasting induces several changes in your body that makes it easier to burn fat. It also reduces the production of insulin while increasing the production of the growth hormone and epinephrine to give a metabolic boost to your body.

Intermittent fasting helps you reduce your intake of calories and helps with weight loss. The primary reason why intermittent fasting is an effective weight loss technique is because it reduces your calorie intake. As such there is no calorie restrictions prescribed by this diet. All the different methods of intermittent fasting involve foregoing meals during the periods of fast. Unless you try to compensate for all this by eating more during the eating window, then you will certainly be consuming fewer calories than usual. Intermittent fasting can lead to significant weight loss if you carefully follow the protocols of this diet for at least three weeks. It isn't just fat loss that you will experience on this diet; you will also notice that you are losing fat from your abdominal region. The benefits of intermittent fasting are not restricted to just weight loss. This diet has a positive effect on your metabolic health and also helps prevent any chronic diseases.

You don"t have to necessarily count calories while following any method of intermittent fasting, but you need to maintain a calorie deficit if you want to lose weight. Intermittent fasting helps reduce your calorie intake without setting up any calorie restrictions.

One of the side effects of a diet that helps you lose fat is that it also causes you to burn muscle while burning fat.

When it comes to intermittent fasting, you will not be burning any muscle mass and, in fact, it helps you gain lean muscle mass. The reduction in muscle mass while on intermittent fasting is quite low when compared to a diet that prescribes continuous calorie restriction.

Apart from this, it is also easier to eat healthily while following this diet. The simplicity of this diet is the main reason for all the benefits it offers. You can select any method of intermittent fasting and you will notice that you are eating healthier meals than before. If you want to follow the OMAD protocol, then you can eat only one meal per day. If you can eat only one meal, then you need to make sure that the meal that you eat will fill you up so that you can go through the day without feeling hungry. The foods that will fill you up for longer are foods rich in protein and fiber. So, knowingly or unknowingly you will start to incorporate healthy foods into your diet. For instance, eating a bowl of lettuce will make you feel fuller for longer than a packet of chips. So, you will be making healthier food choices.

At the end of the day, intermittent fasting is a wonderful dieting protocol that you can follow to lose weight. The main reason for weight loss on this diet is the reduction in the intake of calories.

Chapter Three: Improved Health

Intermittent fasting is a wonderful dieting protocol that offers several health benefits. In this section, you will learn about the different ways in which this diet will improve your overall health.

Weight loss

One of the primary benefits of intermittent fasting is weight loss. Intermittent fasting oscillates between periods of eating and fasting. While fasting, your calorie intake reduces naturally and it helps you lose weight and maintain it as well. Apart from that, it also stops you from indulging in any form of mindless eating. Whenever you consume food, your body converts the food into glucose. The glucose that it needs immediately is converted into energy and the rest is stored within the body in the form of fat cells. Not all the food you consume is converted into energy. So, all the unused energy is stored as fat within your cells. When you start to skip meals, your body will reach into its internal stores of energy. Once your body starts to burn fats to provide energy it automatically kick starts the process of weight loss. Also, most of the fat is usually stored in the abdominal region. If you want to lose fat from your abdominal region, then this is the best diet for you.

Sleep

Obesity is rampant these days. In fact, it is a major health problem that humanity is suffering from. The primary cause of obesity apart from terrible lifestyle and food choices is the lack of sleep. Intermittent fasting regulates your circadian rhythm and it encourages better sleep cycle. When your body is sufficiently rested, it is capable of burning fats effectively. A good sleep cycle has several physiological benefits like an increase in your energy levels and an overall improvement in your mood.

Resistance to illnesses

Intermittent fasting assists in the growth as well as the regeneration of cells. Did you know that the human body has an internal mechanism for repairing all the damaged cells? Well, think of it as internal housekeeping that ensures that all the cells in your body are performing optimally. When you follow the protocols of intermittent fasting it improves the overall functioning of your cells. So, it directly helps improve the natural defense mechanism in your body and increases the resistance to diseases as well as illnesses.

A healthy heart

As mentioned in the previous chapter, intermittent fasting promotes weight loss. Burning up all the stored unnecessary fats in the body helps improve your cardiovascular health. The buildup of plaque in the blood vessels is referred to as atherosclerosis. Atherosclerosis occurs when fat deposits start building up in the blood vessels and it is the primary cause of different cardiovascular diseases. Endothelium is a thin lining present in the blood vessels and a dysfunction of this lining causes atherosclerosis. Obesity is one of the main reasons for the build-up of plaque in blood vessels. Stress, as well as inflammation, worsens this problem. Intermittent fasting helps reduce and remove the plaque deposits and helps tackle obesity. So, if you want to improve the health of your heart, then this is the best diet for you.

A healthy gut

Did you know that your gut is the home for several millions of microorganisms? These microorganisms are helpful and are essential for the optimal functioning of the digestive system. These microorganisms are known as microbiome. The gut microbiome is necessary for a healthy gut. A healthy digestive system helps with better absorption of food and improves the functioning of your stomach. So, a simple diet change can help you improve your gut"s health.

Tackles diabetes

Diabetes is a terrible problem. In fact, it is right alongside with obesity as one of the leading health concerns these days. Diabetes is also a primary indicator for the risk in the increase of different cardiovascular diseases like heart attacks and strokes. When the level of glucose is alarmingly high in the bloodstream and there isn't sufficient insulin to process the glucose, it causes diabetes. When the body starts developing a resistance to insulin, it is quite difficult to regulate the sugar levels in the body. Intermittent fasting reduces the problem of insulin sensitivity and effectively helps tackle and manage diabetes.

Reduces inflammation

Whenever your body notices an internal problem, it powers up its natural defense mechanism - inflammation. Inflammation in moderate amounts is desirable and helpful. However, it doesn"t mean that all forms of inflammation are good. Excess inflammation causes various health problems like arthritics, atherosclerosis and neurodegenerative disorders. Any inflammation of this form is known as chronic inflammation. Chronic inflammation is quite painful, and it can restrict your body"s movements.

Promotes cell repair

When you start fasting, the cells in your body engage themselves in the process of waste removal. Waste removal refers to the process of breaking down dysfunctional cells and proteins. This process is known as autophagy and is quintessential for the upkeep of your body. Do you like accumulating waste in your home? Similarly, it is important to ensure that your body doesn"t start collecting any toxic wastes. Autophagy is the natural way of getting rid of all unnecessary things from your body. Autophagy protects the neurons in your brain from any cell degeneration. It not only protects the neurons, but it also prevents them from excitotoxic stress. All this helps the brain replace the damaged cells and replace them with healthy new cells. When your body does this naturally, it improves the health of your brain. Autophagy also increases the lifespan of cells and promotes longevity.

Improves memory

Intermittent fasting also helps improve your ability to learn and retain things. Improving your memory is one of the best protective measures against neurodegenerative diseases. A diet that restricts the intake of calories helps improve your memory.

Reduces depression

Dealing with any mood disorder can be quite tricky. Medication isn"t the only means to deal with such disorders. A healthy diet that doesn"t fill your body with unnecessary calories leads to an overall improvement in mood. Not just mood, but it also improves your mental clarity and promotes alertness.

Chapter Four: Increased Spirituality

Thoth is believed to be the Egyptian God of magic, wisdom, writing and the moon. One of the scriptures of Thoth says, "The Soul is nourished by fire and air, and the body by water and earth."

Up until now, you were learning about the different aspects of intermittent fasting and the various benefits it offers. The increasing research in this field shows that fasting not only helps with physical healing of the body, but it has certain spiritual benefits as well. In fact, fasting has been a part of several spiritual practices since time immemorial. Fasting is not a practice that is exclusive to a single faith. There are several religions across the globe believe in the spiritual role of fasting like Christianity, Buddhism, Taoism, Islam, Jainism, Hinduism and many more.

Fasting is a healing tool that has mental, physical and spiritual benefits. It affects an individual on different plateaus of being. From a physical standpoint, fasting helps with toxin removal and helps offer protection against various diseases. From a mental and emotional standpoint, fasting helps the mind get rid of all unnecessary worries and anxieties. In fact, it also helps overcome certain addictions.

All of these benefits come together and increase exponentially when you take a look at the various spiritual benefits of fasting. Spiritual experience is something that is unique for every person. The way a person experiences the spiritual aspect of fasting differs from one person to the next. One thing that all religions agree to about fasting is that it opens up a person to form a deeper connection with his or her soul and this, in turn, makes them more receptive to forming a deeper connection with a higher power. When you focus our attention on the eternal soul that resides within, you tend to become attuned with all the energy present in the universe and the fact that this energy continuously flows within us.

By taking a break from a physical aspect of life like the consumption of food, it increases your awareness of different sensations that course through your body that you might have otherwise never noticed. The clarity of body, mind and emotions allows your spirit to come alive and it helps you realize different things about yourself, your life and the world present around you. In this section, you will learn about the spiritual symbolism of fasting in different religions and the spiritual benefits of fasting.

Fasting in Different Religions

Fasting in Christianity

In Christianity, it was believed that after John baptized Jesus in the Jordan River, Jesus had fasted for 40 days in the wilderness. The combination of these two events marks the starting point of how he started his ministry as Christ. Moses is believed to have fasted for 40 days and the same is stated in the book of Exodus. In Christianity, the purpose of a fast is to let you focus on God and not on the other materialistic things present in the world. Fasting is a means of forming and strengthening a bond with divinity and the cosmos. It is about willingly giving up your connection and attachment with the physical world of desires and concentrate on something more spiritual.

The teachings of Christianity believe that through fasting you can empower your commitment to God and your spirituality. That it helps you free yourself from the grip that Satan has over you and it opens you up for spiritual revival. It is believed that spiritual fasting helps bring you closer to the Divine being, opens you up to allow miracles into your life and sharpens your sense of spiritual awareness.

Fasting in Buddhism

According to the teachings of Buddhism, Buddha underwent an extreme fast before he received his enlightenment. Buddha believed that fasting allowed him to reach a new height of enlightenment. The scriptures show that Buddha"s fast was so extreme that his eyes dug deep in his skull and he got extremely weak. It was only after he was given a bowl of porridge with milk that he accepted nourishment, and he sat in deep meditation until he attained enlightenment.

According to different Buddhist traditions, fasting is considered to be a means to reach a state of being where the mind is truly at peace regardless of any physical discomforts. In fact, it is believed to bring about inner peace even in an uncomfortable state. Buddhist teachings prescribe the importance of adopting a "middle path"- moderation of food (neither the rejection of food nor consumption in excess). Thus, the duration of the fast is flexible and it differs from one individual to the next.

Fasting in Islam

In Islam, it is believed that Muhammad initiated a method of frequent fasting and it is quite similar to the present-day method of intermittent fasting. It is believed that he used to abstain from drinking or eating anything from sunrise to sunset and did so as a means of prayer to Allah, the Almighty. In Islam, this form of fasting is quite popular during the month of Ramadan. For Muslins across the globe, this is a common method of fasting every year during the holy month of Ramadan. The fast usually lasts the entire month and is considered to be a holy offering to God.

In the Muslim faith, fasting is believed to develop self-restraint, self-discipline and a means of improving one"s manners. Fasting is a spiritual shield that protects an individual from the tempting desires and sinful behaviors of the mortal world. Therefore, it produces a sense of divine equality and the freedom from want in an individual who observes the fasts. This release of the human spirit from the terrible clutches of lust and helps maintain moderation.

Fasting in Jainism

Fasting is a common practice in Jainism and it is quite similar to its eastern counterpart of Buddhism. The teachings of Jainism believe that fasting purifies the body, mind and soul of the individual and guides them on the path of asceticism and renunciation. All this is a result of the teachings of their leader - Mahavir, who spent a lot of his time fasting. According to the teachings of this faith, it is not merely about fasting, but it is about wanting to not eat. If they continue to desire food while fasting it renders the fast pointless.

In Jainism, the idea of fasting is in support to their five vows - the vow of not indulging in violence, the vow of being truthful, the vow of chastity, the vow of non-possession and the vow to not steal. The buildup of toxins in the body prevents the body from being wholesome and pure. So, they believe that fasting helps cleanse the body and mind and returns a person to their natural state of being. The teachings of Jainism are also of the opinion that fasting promotes physical healing of the body.

Fasting in Taoism

According to the religion of Taoism, fasting helps cleanse the body and mind so that a person can be a clearer state of being and have a healthy respect towards the food that nourishes the body. They believe in the simple concept of "garbage in and garbage out," if you eat food that"s junk or consists of animals and plants that were mistreated, then you send your body and mind into a state of mayhem and it disrupts your natural state of being.

According to the Book of Rites, it is said that fasting also helps a person communicate with the spirit world. Fasting is associated with the chanting of religious scriptures. And it is believed that such a practice will reward the individual with good fortune that's a result of the amassing values and virtues of a pure soul. Fasting not only helps save the body from the buildup of undesirable toxins, but it also saves such a person from misfortune. Finally, fasting is also believed to make an individual conscious of his or her food consumption and this, in turn, can help the individual lead a healthy life.

"A genuine fast will cleanse the body, mind and soul. It crucifies the flesh and to that extent it helps set the soul free."- Gandhi

By now you can clearly see that spirituality and fasting go hand in hand. Fasting is an integral part of different faiths and the benefits of fasting are numerous. Ultimately, the experience that one has of fasting will be different from that of others, but a common belief is that it deepens the connection a person has with their soul and the Cosmos.

Fasting in Meditation

Fasting is not only associated with different systems of belief of faith, but it is also a major part of meditation. Deep breathing and expanding one"s awareness are important proponents of meditation and fasting helps achieve all this. When your body doesn"t spend energy on digesting food, your internal mechanisms adapt themselves to it and start processing nutrients from the food you consume previously. After a while, you can easily tap into the way your body feels and you can understand your body rather deeply.

It also helps you understand where different desires come from - whether a desire is a by-product of your ego or if it is a calling from your inner soul. You become aware of all your attachments to food as a means of distraction. It allows you to take control of your spirituality and the desires of the physical world that we live in.

Deep pranamic breathing is an important part of meditation and this practice helps you gain energy. During an extended fast you can feel that your energy levels are decreasing. During such times, if you concentrate on deep breathing, you will feel refreshed and you will understand that the practice of meditation transcends the boundaries for need of food to sustain yourself.

Your intention to start a fast can be physical or spiritual. If the purpose of fasting is to promote physical healing, then you will receive it. If you fast for a spiritual reason, then you will experience the spiritual benefits as well. When you fast, you will experience all the physical, mental and spiritual benefits it offer and you will notice a positive change in your outlook towards life. You will be able to reap all these benefits along with the spiritual ones it offers.

Your body is made of muscles and organs. When you exercise you can condition your muscles. When you fast, you can condition your body. Think of fasting as a form of exercise. It takes a while for you to condition your body and it will not happen overnight. You need to be patient with yourself and you need to give your body sufficient time to get used to the new diet.

Spiritual Benefits

Intermittent fasting is quite popular these days. After decades and decades of health fanatics proclaiming that consuming small meals throughout the day is the key to good health, now they are proclaiming the opposite of it. Limiting the intake of food is a better way to go about transforming your life for the better. In fact, with the rise in the popularity of intermittent fasting, people believe that fasting for at least 16 hours a day improves the physical and mental health of an individual.

According to experts, there are multiple reasons why intermittent fasting is good for one"s health. It helps bring about mental clarity, improves the ability to concentrate, reduces the levels of sugar and improves the health of the heart. You get the idea right? There is plenty of good that comes from fasting. While all these benefits can change your life for the better. There is another aspect of fasting that needs to be given due credit and that"s the effect it has on one"s spirituality. As mentioned in the previous section, there are various religions that believe that fasting is a great way to open up the pathway to spiritual enlightenment.

That being said, there is so much more to fasting than not eating. So, if this concept is new to you, then here are the reasons why you need to incorporate fasting into your life to give your soul a positive nudge.

Strengthens resolve

If you are having any difficulty making a decision or are trying to understand the answer to the ever-present question of "What am I doing with my life?" then including fasting with some form of prayer will give you the answer. It will help you see past all the distractions and will strengthen your resolve. When you deny your body something, even a little bit, you are bound to be more levelheaded and will be mindful. It will put you in a better mental space that helps you get in touch with your spiritual needs and therefore, it will help you make you feel confident about the decisions that you make. Fasting helps to get rid of temptations and when you can do this, you can think better. When you can think better and in a clear manner, it certainly helps you make better decisions. Strengthening your resolve is essential to get through the hurdles of life to attain your goals.

"Fasting is a good shield for the soul, a steadfast companion for the body, a weapon for the valiant and a gymnasium for athletes."- St. Basil.

Instills discipline

Fasting requires a lot of self-discipline. Fasting is the voluntary abstinence from food. You need to discipline your mind to stop it from thinking about food when you are fasting. Self-discipline and self-control are often used synonymously. However, they aren"t synonyms, not in the strict sense. Restraint is essential for self-discipline and self-discipline to improve self-control. Does that sound confusing? Well, it is quite simple. Only when you have a little self-control will you be able to control your impulses and not give into random whims. When you can focus and not get distracted, you can develop your self-discipline. If you are self-disciplined, you are bound to have a high level of self-control. So, these two concepts are dependent on one another. When you control your thoughts and impulses you can focus on the important things in life. Self-discipline is an important tool that you can use in all aspects of your life.

Humble

The world that we live in is full of distractions. In fact, most of us have the world at our fingertips and it can at times make you feel like a god. Doesn't it make you feel quite powerful that you can communicate with someone who lives across the world from you? Within a couple of swipes, you can purchase something that you want, and you can even tell others about it. Think of fasting as an antidote to all the power that we experience these days. It helps you remind about the frail nature of the human beings. After all, humans are nothing but a speck in the universe. When you remind yourself of your frailty, it helps you bring closer to God.

Closer to God

Fasting helps open up the spiritual gateway to the Cosmos. When you make a sacrifice, regardless of whether it is big or not, it brings you closer to God. It helps you connect with the cosmos on a spiritual sphere. Only when you give up something do you realize that you love something. Sacrifice, even if it"s temporary, is the best way to understand what you love.

Well, if you want to reap all these spiritual benefits, then all that you need to do is get started with intermittent fasting.

Chapter Five: Getting More Work Done

Intermittent fasting is a great way to improve your productivity. This diet not only helps improve your overall health, but it will also make you quite productivity. In this section, you will learn about the different ways in which intermittent fasting will make you productive and the simple tips that you can follow to ease the fasting period.

Become more Productive

Don't have to think about food

Regardless of whether we do it consciously or not, most of us tend to keep thinking about what the next meal will be. When you spend so much of your time thinking about what you will eat, you are essentially wasting your time. For instance, let us assume that you take about four coffee breaks while at work and each break lasts for about 15 minutes. So, you are wasting about 60 minutes of your day being absolutely unproductive. When you are fasting, you can use this time to do something else. When you eliminate the need for food, it gives you an opportunity to be more productive. Not just that, it also helps you focus on the task at hand instead of worrying about other distractions.

Better energy levels

People tend to believe that fasting for extended periods of time will make them feel weak or even sluggish. Well, that"s certainly not the case with intermittent fasting. When you are following the protocols of this diet, you condition your body to start burning its internal reserves of fat to provide energy. Once your body starts to do this, then you will have a constant supply of energy throughout the day. So, even when you don"t eat, your body will keep burning fats to provide energy. Usually, you notice a sudden dip in your energy at around 4-5 in the evening. This happens because your body is used to burning glucose to provide energy and the lack of it will make you hungry. However, when you start following intermittent fasting, you will not notice any sudden dips in your energy levels and you will feel quite energetic throughout the day.

Discipline

Self-discipline is important for fasting. Self-discipline improves your productivity. When you know the things that you must focus on, you can get them done on time. Instead of whiling away your time on unnecessary activities, you can concentrate and improve your overall productivity. Not just that, it will even make you happy. Self-discipline ensures that you can get the right things done at the right time. All this will make you a happier individual. A person with self-discipline does have more time in a day than others. It doesn"t mean that you will get extra hours in a day. It merely means that you have more time to do all the extra work when you don"t procrastinate.

It helps you decide what is right and what is wrong. It helps you to distinguish between good and bad habits. Not just separate, but it even provides you the necessary willpower to do the right thing. If you get sufficient rest, nutrition, and exercise, your overall health will improve. Self-Discipline will help you in to stay healthy.

Additional Tips

Getting sufficient sleep

Getting sufficient sleep will not only keep you healthy, but will make you happier as well. The age-old saying "Early to bed, early to rise makes a man healthy, wealthy, and wise" is true. Make sure that you sleep early and get about 7-8 hours of undisturbed sleep. If you cannot wake up on your own in the morning, then you can set an alarm. Give yourself an hour to unwind before going to bed. You can read a book, watch some TV, go for a walk, or do anything that will relax you. It isn"t just about the number of hours you sleep for, but the quality of sleep that matters as well. Here are a couple of simple tips that will help you in getting better sleep at night.

Set aside 8 hours for sleeping and create a sleep schedule for yourself. Go to bed and wake up at the same time every day. Try to be as consistent as possible. If you aren"t able to sleep within 20 minutes of lying on the bed, leave your bedroom and do something soothing. Then go back to bed when you feel tired. After a while your body will get conditioned to the sleep schedule.

Don"t get to bed when you are feeling hungry or after eating a lot. Avoid large and heavy meals before your bedtime. Physical discomfort will prevent you from sleeping. Nicotine, caffeine, and alcohol must be consumed with caution, especially before sleeping. These three substances can wreak havoc on your sleep.

Your bedroom must be cool, dark, and quiet. The room must be restful and conducive of sleeping. You cannot possibly fall asleep in a room with harsh lighting, loud music, and the wrong temperature.

If you like to take a nap during the day, try to limit it as much as you possibly can. Even when you do take a nap, don"t let it exceed 30 minutes.

Develop a bedtime routine for yourself like taking a bath, reading a book, or listening to music before going to sleep. Familiarity creates a routine and there"s comfort in routine.

Regular physical activity helps in sleeping better. However, don"t indulge in any tiring physical activity right before going to sleep. If your body is full of adrenaline and endorphins, you won"t be able to sleep.

Don"t contemplate about your worries late at night. Don"t let your stress get to you. Learn to manage your stress. You will learn more about this in this chapter.

Eating healthy foods

Avoid all sorts of processed foods that are full of sugars, unhealthy fats, and undesirable carbs. Instead, opt for healthy foods that are rich in fiber, nutrients and the essential macros. Healthy food will nourish your body and will leave you feeling energetic. Unhealthy foods like chocolates or chips can be replaced with some fruit or nuts. Here are a couple of simple tips that you can keep in mind to make sure that you are eating wholesome food.

Have complex carbohydrates like whole grains and leafy vegetables instead of starchy foods like bread, pasta or pizza. Your meal must be rich in protein because it not only leaves you feeling fuller for longer, but it is good for you as well. Stay away from all processed foods and instead opt for healthy treats like kale chips, nuts, fruit, or anything that isn"t full of saturated fats and trans fats. Replace sugary drinks with water (sparkling or still). Create a food plan for yourself. If you are interested in cooking, then learn to experiment with recipes and cook something different. Healthy food doesn"t mean bland salads, so keep an open mind and try your hand at cooking. If you plan your meals in advance, then you can do all the meal prep on your day off, this does simplify the entire cooking process.

Drink plenty of water

Water is good for your body and drinking plenty of water will make your skin clearer and will flush out all the toxins from your body. Make it a habit to have at least 8 glasses of water daily. If you want to, you can add some flavorings or electrolytes to your water to spruce it up. Slices of lemon, different berries, a handful of mint leaves, or slices of cucumber can be added to water for making detox water. By following these five simple tips, you can trick yourself into drinking water.

Drinking water needs to be convenient. Carry a water bottle or a sipper with you wherever you go. If a water bottle is handy, it is more likely that you will drink water without a reminder. Instead of sugary sodas and sweetened beverages, you can have unsweetened water-based drinks. Instead of a Frappuccino, have a cup of Americano. Make it a point to drink a glass of water before and after your meals. Set a goal and measure the amount of water you are drinking daily. If you keep a track of your water intake, you will be motivated to drink more. Don"t forget to drink water even when you go out drinking with your friends. Don"t let your body get dehydrated.

Learn to manage stress

Stress can take away your happiness. You need to learn to manage stress and not let it get to you. Stress complicates things and it hinders your ability to think clearly and retards your productivity as well. Here are a couple of steps that you can follow for managing your stress.

Avoid caffeine, alcohol, and nicotine because these will just make you feel more stressed and they aren"t good for your health. Caffeine and nicotine and stimulating agents, therefore they will just increase your stress instead of decreasing it. Alcohol is a depressant and too much of it will make you feel more stressed than usual

Stress increases the production of adrenaline and cortisol. These hormones are responsible for our "fight or flight" instinct. Physical exercise helps in normalizing these hormones. Not just that, physical exercise produces endorphins that will improve your overall mood and make you happier.

The importance of good sleep is paramount. You cannot function effectively and efficiently if you don"t get sufficient rest. Your body needs some time to reboot its functions and recharge itself. Don"t burn yourself out and give your body the rest it deserves.

You can reduce your stress by talking to someone about it. You don"t have to go to a psychologist. Just talk to someone who can listen to you. When you share your stress with someone else, it does get better and a situation will not seem intimidating. You might even get a solution to solving your problem by discussing it with someone.

Stop Overeating

You need to have well-balanced meals. Eat only when you are hungry and stop yourself from eating unnecessarily. Here are a couple of simple things that you can do to avoid overeating.

Learn to eat slowly. This certainly isn't a new concept, but not many follow it. We are all in a hurry these days. Take a moment and slow down. Take a sip of water between bites and chew your food thoroughly before swallowing it. Don't just gulp your food learn to chew it slowly. **Start paying attention to what you are eating.** Savor the food you are eating and don't just stuff yourself with food. Think about the different textures and flavors. Savor every bite you eat and make it a pleasurable experience. Make your first bites count and satisfy your taste buds. **Make use of a smaller plate**, this will enable you to control the portions you eat. Stay away from foods that are rich in calories but do nothing to satisfy your appetite. Choose foods that will fill you up; foods that are satisfying. Foods rich in protein and fiber will fill your tummy. **Instead of having a bar of chocolate or a pint of ice cream, have a portion of meat with grilled vegetables.** This will satiate your hunger. Foods that are rich in calories make you feel full for a while and you will be hungry within an hour. This leads to overeating. By being mindful of what you are eating, you can stop yourself from overeating. While eating, make it a point to stay away from all electronic gadgets. This means no television. The next time you are bored, don"t reach for the box of cookies or the bag of chips. Think before indulging in mindless eating.

Slow down

Did you know that it takes your brain a minimum of 20 minutes to register that you are feeling full. So, eat slowly and your brain will be able to register when you are full. You can slow down by following a very simple technique that is referred to as fork down. This will help you in enjoying your meal and eat slowly as well. It is quite simple to follow. Take smaller bites of food that you usually do and put that morsel in your mouth. Put down your fork, spoon, chopsticks or your choice of cutlery on the table and release it from your hand. Let your hands be free while you are chewing. This act of putting your fork down (quite literally) prevents you from prepping the next bite even before swallowing your last one. Now, chew your food and chew it well. Notice the texture and the taste of what you are eating. Softer food must be chewed for 5-10 times and harder or denser foods up to 30 times before you swallow it. After chewing, swallow your food completely. Once you have swallowed it, pick up your fork and reload it for your next bite. Then repeat this process all over again. Continue this technique throughout the duration of your meal. You will notice that the time spent eating will increase and you will feel fuller earlier than usual.

When you feel full, stop eating. Don"t eat just for the sake of eating or because there"s food left.

Keep track of your weight

Start keeping a track of your weight and weigh yourself daily. This will help you in keeping a tab on your overall fitness and also assist you in identifying any changes in your weight quite easily. Your weight won't stay constant and slight fluctuations are likely. Your weight can fluctuate due to the recent meal you had, level of hydration, exercise pattern, and your menstrual cycle as well. Always weigh yourself first thing in the morning since this will provide you with a more realistic picture of your weight. You must be consistent in doing so. For all those who are tech savvy, you can track your weight by making use of several applications. There are plenty of paid and free mobile applications to choose from that will help you in keeping a track of your weight and provide you with the necessary statistics. If you are more old school, then you can maintain a diary for tracking your weight. Make it a habit to weigh yourself, but don't start obsessing about your weight. It is not just your weight that you must keep a track of, but your body measurements as well. At times, your weight might stay the same, but your measurements can differ. This will also help you in tracking your weight loss.

Eat rainbows

The best way to ensure that you have a healthy diet that provides you with all the necessary vitamins and nutrients that your body needs is by making sure that you are eating the rainbow. Yes, you read it correctly and don't take it literally. This simply means that you must include vegetables and fruit of different colors in your daily diet to improve your overall health.

Red colored foods have lycopene, an antioxidant that provides you with a burst of energy and also helps in reducing your risk of cancer. The food-list includes red peppers, tomatoes, apples, cherries, grapes, strawberries, raspberries, and watermelon. Orange colored foods contain beta-carotene (vitamin A). Foods like carrots, pumpkin, peppers, oranges, tangerines, nectarines, sweet potatoes and yams are good for your eyes. Yellow foods are rich in carotenoids and lutein that help in improving your eyesight and prevent cancer. Have a portion of yellow colored foods like peppers, cantaloupe, beans, zucchini, squash, grapefruit, lemon, and papayas. Green colored foods contain flavonoids that improve the functioning of the brain, memory, and the cardiovascular health of an individual. Have lots of green leafy vegetables and anything that's green in color. Blue and purple colored foods also have flavonoids and include blueberries, nightshades like eggplant and peppers, red cabbage and grapes. White colored foods like cauliflower, garlic, peas, potatoes, bananas, and pears contain selenium and allicin that are good for the heart.

Keeping your portions in check

You must start keeping a track of the portions you eat. This will also help in making sure that you are having a well-balanced meal. Your calorie intake must be less than the calories you are burning. If it isn"t, then your body will simply start storing the remaining calories in the form of fat cells and you will gain weight. You don"t need a set of measuring cups and a measuring scale for keeping an eye on the portions you consume. You can measure the portions by using your hand. Yes, it is quite simple and regardless of where you are, you will always be able to check the portion size.

As a rule of thumb, men will need two portions and women will need just one. Your palm signifies the amount of protein you must eat. The recommended amount of meat in a meal is about 3 ounces or the size and weight of a deck of cards. Your palm without including your fingers is close to this size. The amount of vegetable that you must include in a meal is equivalent to your clenched fist. Now, cup your hand and that"s the amount of carbs that you must have in a meal. Carbs can be obtained from pastas, breads, and even starchy veg like potatoes. Fats must be equivalent to the size of your thumb. That"s approximately the size of a tablespoon. For measuring the portion of cheese, make use of your fingers. A portion of cheese must be roughly equivalent to two of your fingers placed together.

So, to sum it all up, a piece of meat that fits into your palm, a fistful of vegetables, a cupped hand of carbs, your thumb represents the portion of fat and your fingers for the portion of cheese. If you have three to four meals a day by making use of the above-mentioned portions, then you will be having a well-balanced meal.

Chapter Six: Success Stories

A good diet is all that you need to turn your life around. You don"t need powerful and expensive medicines to better your life. You merely need to be mindful of what you eat and when you eat, and Janielle Wright"s story will reinforce this belief.

Janielle Wright is a health and a beauty influencer who weighed 337 lbs. before following the protocols of intermittent fasting. Her body used to be in constant pain and she even had trouble breathing at night. She used to go to sleep worrying that she might not wake up in the morning. Her worries weren"t restricted to her health, the 28-year old mother was worried that she will never get to see her daughter, Noah, grow up. She was tired of all the fad diets that promised quick results. All such diets did her no good and only made it worse for her health. In January 2018, she decided to try intermittent fasting. By restricting her eating window and eating only during the feeding window, she managed to lose over 65 pounds.

Wright chose a method of intermittent fasting that restricted her eating window to about 8 hours and she was essentially fasting for the other 16 hours. She scheduled her diet such that her first meal was at noon and her last meal at around 8 p.m. She was eating only two meals per day and was avoiding snacking between her meals. She stuck to low-carb meals and her daily calorie intake was between 1800 to 2000 calories per day. She used MyFitnessPal app to track her calorie intake.

She wanted to change, and she wanted to do something to not just lose weight but improve her overall health as well. Intermittent fasting addressed all her concerns and really helped her turn her life around.

The one thing about intermittent fasting that Wright enjoys is the fact that it doesn"t place any restrictions on the kind of foods you can, as long as you avoid junk food. A consistent exercise routine and piously following the diet helped her drop over 65 pounds in less than six months. About 15 minutes of warm-up cardio and 30 minutes of intensive exercising six days a week helped speed up her weight loss. She says consistency is the key. She loved her experience with intermittent fasting so much that she believes she can sustain her new diet even in the long run. Being constant, consistent and patient are the three things she believes helped her achieve her weight loss and fitness goals.

If she can do it, then so can you!

If Wright"s store inspired you, here is another story that will certainly want you to get started with your diet today!

Dwayne managed to drop 52 lbs. in seven months. He is just like you, a normal guy, with a happy family, who likes his work and is happy in general. Everything was great in his life except for the fact that he was overweight and needed a good diet that will help him lose weight in a healthy manner. While looking for the "perfect" diet, he stumbled across intermittent fasting and there was no looking back for him since then. Dwayne claims that following the diet for seven months has made him feel like he is a new person altogether. The diet has made him change his unhealthy eating habits and has helped him lead a healthier life. He claims that intermittent fasting coupled with nutritious meals and a little exercise have helped him not only lose weight but make him feel quite energetic as well. Apart from this, the diet has also improved his mental clarity and overall productivity.

Intermittent fasting is also quite popular among Hollywood celebrities. Several celebrities like Hugh Jackman, Terry Crews, Beyoncé, Jennifer Lopez, Nicole Kidman and Ben Affleck swear by this diet. So, if you want to look like your favorite celebrity, then all that you need to do is start following the diet that helps them retain their good

Conclusion

I want to thank you once again for purchasing this book. I hope it proved to be an entertaining and an informative read.

Intermittent fasting is a wonderful diet that is quite different from all the traditional diets. It is quite simple to follow this dynamic diet. You merely need to select an eating window for yourself and you are good to go. As long as you eat only during the eating window and fast throughout the day, you will be able to see a positive change in your life within no time. While following this diet, you need to be patient with yourself and keep an open mind.

Now, that you are aware of all the different aspects of this diet along with the benefits it offers, the next step is to get started as soon as you can. If you are ready to turn your life around and achieve your weight loss and fitness goals, then OMAD is the diet for you! So, go ahead, take the first step to turning your life around!

Thank you and all the best!

Resources

https://www.healthline.com/nutrition/intermittent-fasting-and-weight-loss

https://blog.bulletproof.com/intermittent-fasting-benefits/

http://grottonetwork.com/keep-the-faith/belief/spiritual-benefits-of-intermittent-fasting/

https://www.thriveglobal.com/stories/how-fasting-absolutely-skyrocketed-my-productivity/

https://www.dietdoctor.com/intermittent-fasting/success-stories/all